Thomas came to Daisy empty-handed after giving out bedding to their exhausted neighbors.

"Is there anything left for me or should I curl up in the bath for the night?" Daisy was only half joking. As much as she was longing for a bed, she would sleep anywhere right now.

"I thought you could sleep in my room."

Her eyebrows shot up at the presumption. "Excuse me?"

Thomas at least looked embarrassed when she queried his proposition. "I mean, you can take the bed. I'll take the floor. I know I should give up my room for someone else, but I'm not ready to leave strangers alone with my personal items."

There was a warm glow inside her at the thought he was happy for her to have entry into his inner sanctum. He no longer saw her as an unwanted stranger.

"In that case, take me to your bed, your lordship." She could not help but tease him when he looked so adorably ruffled. Up until now she had not seen him as anything other than confident and cool in his actions.

Dear Reader,

There is nothing like writing about two broken souls who don't know how much they need one another and watching them fight the inevitable. I do enjoy torturing my characters so their happy ending is all that more sweeter!

Daisy and Thomas have both been scarred by the past and are grieving in their own way for the man who inadvertently brought them together. Neither is prepared to budge an inch to make room for someone else in their lives, but Mother Nature has other ideas. A flood, lots of drama and being forced to stay together mean they have no choice but to admit they are more than work colleagues.

It's a rocky road to love for the couple but one I hope you enjoy taking with them. I promise, it's all worth it in the end!

Happy reading!

Karin xx

A GP TO
STEAL HIS HEART

—

KARIN BAINE

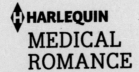

HARLEQUIN
MEDICAL
ROMANCE

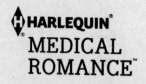

HARLEQUIN®
MEDICAL ROMANCE™

Recycling programs for this product may not exist in your area.

ISBN-13: 978-1-335-40927-0

A GP to Steal His Heart

Copyright © 2022 by Karin Baine

For questions and comments about the quality of this book, please contact us at CustomerService@Harlequin.com.

Harlequin Enterprises ULC
22 Adelaide St. West, 41st Floor
Toronto, Ontario M5H 4E3, Canada
www.Harlequin.com

Printed in U.S.A.

Karin Baine lives in Northern Ireland with her husband, two sons and her out-of-control notebook collection. Her mother and her grandmother's vast collection of books inspired her love of reading and her dream of becoming a Harlequin author. Now she can tell people she has a *proper* job! You can follow Karin on Twitter, @karinbaine1, or visit her website for the latest news—karinbaine.com.

Books by Karin Baine

Harlequin Medical Romance

Pups that Make Miracles
Their One-Night Christmas Gift

Single Dad Docs
The Single Dad's Proposal

Midwife Under the Mistletoe
Their One-Night Twin Surprise
Healed by Their Unexpected Family
Reunion with His Surgeon Princess
One Night with Her Italian Doc
The Surgeon and the Princess
The Nurse's Christmas Hero
Wed for Their One Night Baby

Visit the Author Profile page
at Harlequin.com for more titles.

For Paddy, who never let the truth
get in the way of a good story xx

CHAPTER ONE

THE FRESH SEA air smelled like freedom. Daisy got out of her car and inhaled a lungful as she stretched out her limbs. She had expected to reach her destination three days ago but her replacement at the clinic had taken ill and Daisy had agreed to stay on to share the workload until another could be found. As a result, the leisurely break before she began her new job had not happened and she would be throwing herself in at the deep end today.

It had been a long drive from London and, exhausted, she had made an overnight stop in a motel to break up the journey rather than risk falling asleep at the wheel. Her last-minute decision meant she had not been able to inform the clinic of her later arrival, but she would still make it on time for her first day.

It would be worth all the trouble to get her own space. Not only was she taking up her new position as a GP in the village of Lit-

tle Morton on the south coast of England
but also she was moving into her own cottage, complete with country garden. A whole
world away from the cramped and stifling
city where she had been working since qual-
ifying. However, before she could enjoy this
new country life she literally had to check
in at the medical practice for a pass into the
village.

Little Morton was privately owned by the
same Earl who had awarded her the scholarship which got her through medical school
and away from her controlling ex at the time.

Since training as a GP she had worked hard
to keep her independence. Though they had
never met in person, she had kept in touch
with the Earl of Morton through emails and
video calls. Through her brief, unsatisfactory
relationships, he had been her one constant.
Her most recent partner, Ed, had called her a
workaholic, accused her of not enjoying life.
Although she had not mourned his loss when
their relationship had ended, his words had
stayed with her.

Her abusive past had left her afraid to trust
anyone enough to get serious, but she wondered if she had let that influence other as-
pects of her life too. Gradually, she had begun
to see the truth in Ed's words and realised

she made very little time for herself. The fast pace of city life had made it acceptable but, when she had taken a good look, it was obvious she had no real friends or roots. Not 'belonging' anywhere made her worried that one day she would come to regret the decisions she had made and begin to yearn for something new.

When the Earl had told her he was retiring and that his medical practice was in need of someone like her, Daisy thought it the perfect opportunity to start over, as well as finally getting to thank him in person. Yet her arrival was tinged with sadness, with news of the Earl's death coming only weeks before completing her move here. They would never get to meet after all.

The village was every bit as beautiful as she had imagined. Higgledy-piggledy old houses marched down the cobbled street to meet the sea, history evident in every whitewashed wall and timber frame. The vibrant splash of pink and purple dahlias and violet agapanthus bursting from hanging baskets and window boxes welcomed her.

She locked her car and began her walk down the rocky street. In order to maintain the village's original features, only residents were apparently permitted to drive past the town sign. Yet to obtain her status as a local she had to get a parking permit from the medical centre.

The quirkiness of the crowded Elizabethan buildings made her smile, and she could see why traffic was more than an aesthetic issue. Any more than two cars at once here would block the whole road. Yes, Daisy thought, Little Morton was exactly where she needed to be to start her new life.

The medical centre was easy enough to find, a converted old school house which was signposted at the bottom of the hill overlooking the harbour. She thought of the lucky children who had once attended and the fun they must have had down on the shore during sunny days such as today.

As a child she had missed out on simple things like visits to the beach because her stepfather didn't include her in any family outings. Although she'd taken part in swimming lessons provided by the school, an incident in the pool when she had taken cramp in her leg and nearly drowned left her fearful around water.

Something which had not been helped by Aaron, her abusive ex, who found her phobia funny and had pushed her into a pool on a rare holiday together. That panicky feeling of gasping for air while he watched her, laughing, was always at the back of her mind. Along with the notion that if she got into difficulty in the water no one would come to help her.

However, as part of her new life here she thought about working through those fears. If she was brave enough perhaps she could learn to swim here with some support. It would be a shame to live in such a picturesque seascape and not enjoy something as simple as paddling in the shallows.

When she reached the clinic, she ducked under the half-opened shutter and approached the affable-looking lady on the reception desk. 'Eunice? It's me, Daisy. I just need to get the keys for my cottage and a pass so I can get my car in and out of the village before I start work.'

Daisy had spoken to the practice manager on the phone lots of times, but this was their first meeting in person. From everything she had gathered, Eunice had been the Earl's right-hand woman at the clinic. She had even set up video calls between Daisy and her benefactor so they could see each other while they chatted about everything from complicated medical cases they had worked on to their favourite TV shows. It was Eunice who had suggested the online interview which had sealed her position here in Little Morton and Daisy was thankful to know at least one person in the village.

'Daisy? We were expecting you yesterday.' Eunice rushed around from behind her desk and wrapped her in a friendly hug.

'Yes, sorry. I got stuck in traffic and I was so tired I decided it would be safer to check myself into a hotel for the night.'

'No problem. You're here now and I'm sure we have time for a cuppa and a catch-up before we start the clinic.' She took Daisy by the arm and began to guide her towards the back of the building.

'I still have to unpack my stuff at the cottage…' Daisy began to protest but was manoeuvred into a chair in the staffroom, where Eunice set about making that cup of tea.

'That can wait. I'm sure you are dying for a cuppa and I want to hear all about you. I know about the scholarship, of course. Daniel mentioned you'd had a bit of trouble in the past and that was what had set you on the path to medical school.' Eunice had her back to Daisy as she poured water into two cups, unable to see her raised eyebrows.

She was not prepared for someone to be so openly curious about her personal life after living in the city, where most people kept themselves to themselves. But this was the country and Daisy supposed she would have to get used to people in this close-knit community being interested in her background. Even if it was not the most comfortable subject for her to discuss with anyone.

'Er...yes. I was in a difficult relationship. Aaron was...controlling. The Earl's scholarship enabled me to strike out on my own.' It was disconcerting talking about her painful past with a virtual stranger when she did not tend to open up to anyone, but she could already tell Eunice was a kind soul who simply wanted to make her feel at home. Perhaps it was that empathy which drove her to spill more about her troubles.

'You must have been a good student before that though to even get into medical school.' Eunice handed Daisy one of the cups and sat down in the chair next to her, ready to hear the rest of her story.

'I was when I was younger.' School had been her source of stability and the one place she could earn praise for all of her hard work. As a result she had become one of the top students but that had only earned sneering from her stepfamily, who did not like her to get 'above her station'. Despite her detractors Daisy had planned to go to medical school to make something of herself. Then she had met Aaron.

It was not surprising that she had found herself in the thrall of a domineering, manipulative man after the upbringing she'd had. Once her mother had run out and left her with her stepfather and stepbrothers, she had bent over backwards to keep them happy lest she got kicked out of the house.

They had taken advantage, treating her more like a servant than family. Her days had been taken up with chores and looking after them, leaving her no time for a life of her own. She'd swapped that prison for one with a partner who thought a woman's place was in the home, and who was she to disagree when he was the sole breadwinner?

'My partner didn't want me to further my education because he preferred to have me at home in a more "traditional" role.' Which invariably meant tied to the house and not allowed out unaccompanied because he was so paranoid she would cheat on him. It was that stifling behaviour which had made her question her life with Aaron and realise the way he was treating her had nothing to do with love.

When control had turned to violence, that was when she had known it was time to get out.

'Uh huh. I can guess the type. I have daughters of my own and not every boyfriend I have met has been ideal. Thankfully, they're both happily married now so I don't have to worry about them any more in that respect.'

'That's good. It's not easy to meet the right man. Unknown to Aaron, I joined an online support group for women in a similar position to me. That's where I learned about the Earl's scholarship and the rest is history.' Once they had got to know each other better, Daisy had shared some of the details about her background with the Earl. She had no idea if he had told Eunice any of her story, but it was helping them to bond now as they got to know one another. With the Earl gone, Daisy needed as many friends as she could get.

'He was very fond of you. I think he saw you as the daughter he never had.' Eunice's blue eyes filled with tears and Daisy could see theirs had been a special relationship too.

'He was certainly very kind. A real role model for me.' There had not been a supportive male presence in her life until Daisy had received his financial assistance and she liked to think of him as her surrogate father. The one she would have liked to have growing up, instead of the emotionally abusive stepfather she'd had throughout her childhood.

'You and Thomas should get on well. He's very like his father: good with his patients and always puts the job first. I'm sure the two of you have a lot in common. He has been through a lot too and I'm sure he will enjoy having some company around the place.'

'I'm looking forward to meeting him.' It would be a connection to the Earl again and Daisy hoped they might bring each other some comfort when they were both grieving the recent loss of a wonderful man.

'Of course, Thomas inherited his father's title along with the medical practice and the village. He's our new Earl now.'

Daisy could not help thinking those were some big shoes to fill.

'Thanks for the tea and chat, Eunice, but I should really get moving. I've got a busy day ahead of me.' Daisy got up and poured what was left of her tea down the sink. She did not want to get used to lazing around before a shift. Especially when she had so much to do now she was three days behind schedule.

Eunice took an envelope out of her trouser

pocket. 'Okay, there are your keys and your pass. Just wave it in front of the barrier and you can come and go as you please. Soon you'll feel like you've always been here.' She gave Daisy a wink.

'Hopefully it won't be too long before I'm considered a local.' Daisy laughed a little too loudly, suddenly wondering if she would be accepted at all.

At that unfortunate moment a man dressed in a navy three-piece suit walked into the room. Well over six feet, it was easy for him to look down on her five feet four inches, one eyebrow raised as he caught the end of the conversation. The new Earl, she presumed, as she stuck her hand out.

'Daisy Swift. The new GP. Pleased to meet you.'

The tall, unsmiling man looked at her outstretched hand for several moments before shaking it, as though he was worried he might catch something from her. It was difficult not to compare the two Ryan men when on first impressions they appeared to be complete opposites. He did not have the same smiling, ruddy-cheeked face as his father, who had always put her in mind of a Father Christmas figure. Junior had more of a Grinch vibe going on.

'Thomas Ryan. Dr Thomas Ryan, senior partner.' He had that air of superiority and dismissive tone that meant Daisy would have guessed he was the heir apparent even if she had not been told. The Earl never had any airs or graces when they had spoken but Daisy would not have been surprised if Thomas had insisted that everyone addressed him as 'Sir' and decreed no one should make direct eye contact with him.

Nevertheless, Daisy owed a lot to his family and she reminded herself that this was a man in mourning for his father. Dr Ryan Senior had been nothing but sweet to her and she held onto that last ember of hope that Thomas had inherited some of his father's warm nature along with his estate.

'I was very sorry to hear about your father.'

Thomas gave a curt, unemotional nod. 'Your office is next to mine. You'll want to get yourself acquainted with your patient list before your first appointment.' He glanced at his expensive watch as he began to walk away.

Daisy assumed he meant her to follow, but he had not actually welcomed her or acknowledged he knew anything about her arrival. It was such a hefty blow, realising the cheery offspring of her saviour she had dreamed she would be working with in her perfect new job was, in reality, as unwelcoming as the closed barrier to the village. Everything about him shouted, *Stay away. You're not wanted here.*

'I didn't think we opened for another hour or so and I've just arrived. I have my pass now; I'll head to the cottage, throw my belongings inside and come straight back.' She got the distinct impression she had already screwed up before actually doing any work.

He stopped and spun around so suddenly she almost ran into him. 'You mean you haven't even moved in yet? Anyone with an ounce of sense would have come here at least a day early to get settled in. Not try to do it when they're about to start their first day of work.'

'It's not as though I have very far to travel.' Daisy bristled at his tone and criticism. It wakened that need to defend herself hedge-hog-style, where her prickles were deployed to repel any potential predators. She could have told him the reason for her delayed arrival, as she had done with Eunice, but since he had not given her the opportunity to explain before chastising her she was entitled to bite back. Besides, she had still made it here on time ready to work so it shouldn't be a big deal. He didn't know her duty to her patients

was always at the forefront of her mind, but
she would certainly let him know. Along with
the fact she did not take orders from anyone.

Dr Ryan checked his watch again and
huffed out an exasperated breath. All this exchange was missing was an eye roll and she
would feel about two foot high.

'Dr Swift, I'm not sure about the way
you're used to working but our patients, the
residents of Little Morton, have certain standards.' The way he looked her up and down
suggested her appearance alone did not meet
acceptable requirements. By starting off on
the wrong foot, it seemed he was going to
pick over every aspect of her appointment
here.

Daisy would have been apologetic over her
less than satisfactory timing if it wasn't for
his haughty attitude. As it was, she felt the
need to give him a taste of his own medi-
cine so he would realise she was no pushover.
Those days were long gone.

'I'm used to working in a very busy city
surgery, above and beyond normal hours, with
people from all walks of life, and I've never
had any complaints. If Little Morton's high
standards entail starting work earlier than
I've been contracted for, I will take note for
future reference. Now, in order for me to get

back in suitable time for the patients, it might be provident if I have an extra pair of hands.' Daisy folded her arms and waited for his response to her frankly brazen request. It was a risky move, but she had dealt with domineering men her whole life and had finally figured out the best way to deal with them was to stand her ground. To stay strong and not cave in to demands. That did not mean her heart wasn't pounding as she waited for his response.

With another long breath, he began to stalk back the way they'd come, leaving an openmouthed Eunice behind. It was difficult to tell if her shock at the exchange was because of Thomas's rudeness, after she had sung his praises, or because of Daisy's sharp retort. Either way, their personality clash did not bode well for their future working environment.

She wondered what it was about her that had apparently brought out the worst in Dr Ryan when Eunice had been extolling the virtues of the new Earl to her. This was not the kindly man Daisy had been expecting to meet. Okay, so she was a little later than expected but she was here. There was something in his attitude towards her that made her think his problem with her was about more than her delayed arrival. Perhaps he did not appreciate women who stood up for themselves and refused to be browbeaten. Whatever it was, it irked her until she could not resist one last jibe.

'You might want to leave the jacket and waistcoat behind. It wouldn't do for you to get them dirty before clinic starts. How on earth would that look to your discerning patients?'

He unbuttoned his waistcoat and stripped off his outer layers. Hopefully Dr Ryan had got the memo she was not going to be bossed around as though she were a second-class citizen. She might have relied on his father's generosity to get her to this point in her life but she had earned the right to be treated as an equal in their place of work. If he continued to forget that she would simply have to keep reminding him.

Daisy Swift was everything Thomas had feared she would be—loud, obnoxious and unwilling to adapt. The village deserved better in their GP. This was his father's doing but now he was gone Thomas had no one to voice his reservations to any more.

There had been dozens of scholarship recipients over the years who had received his father's help to further their education and career prospects. Most of whom had expressed their gratitude at the time by way of phone calls or gifts, the occasional update in a Christmas card. Daisy was the only one who had become a seemingly permanent feature in his father's life. It had made Thomas question her motives for remaining in contact with an elderly man she had never met. Especially recently, when she had decided to come and live in Little Morton to be closer to him.

There had to be more to her interest in his father than his witty repartee for a young, attractive woman to come all this way, giving up her life in London to do so. Was it his money? Did she think there was something for her in the will? Now his father had passed away, was Thomas her latest target? Too bad for her if she thought he could be sweet-talked when he was still in mourning for a father who had been taken from him by the last duplicitous woman to cross their paths. It was only natural for Thomas to be wary of another stranger in the village, given past events.

His own mother had been a city girl here on holiday when she had caught his father's eye. From what he'd gathered, they had been madly in love for a while, at least on his father's part. When Thomas had been about six years old it seemed his mother had grown tired of life in the village and her family. In typical cliché fashion, she had run off with the gardener after emptying their joint bank account. Thank goodness his father had kept money from his investments in a separate account of his own or she might have cleaned him out entirely. Thomas had not seen or heard from her since and had few memories of her to be over-emotional about the loss.

It was testament to his father's strength of character that the betrayal had not stopped him reaching out to strangers less fortunate than himself. He had offered Thomas's mother a lifeline when he had come along, their union giving her the financial means to escape poverty and the rundown council estate she had been living in. Thomas suspected he had carried on the tradition through his charity work because he had seen the difference money could make in someone else's life. He had tried to get his father to rein in the amount of money he gave away to good causes, through fear that people were taking advantage of him, but helping others had seemed to make the old man happy.

In an effort to recreate that for himself, Thomas had set up his own charitable arm providing monetary assistance to local single parent families who were finding things tough. It was there that he had met Jade, a confident, attractive volunteer whose company he had enjoyed. Unfortunately, their short relationship had apparently provided her criminal associates with the necessary information to burgle the family home when Thomas had been out of town.

The betrayal had been painful, but not as much as watching his parent's health decline after the robbery. Tied up and beaten, he had been left a shell of a man who no longer felt safe in his own home. It was the guilt of being the one who had brought these people into the village which Thomas had struggled with, on top of his grief. Now he was expected to work alongside someone else he knew nothing about. Of course he was wary.

Especially when she did not appear to respect him or his station. He wanted this village to be the safe community his father had always intended and that was hard to achieve with a stranger moving in. It was probably Thomas's own fault he knew very little about Daisy; he'd tended to switch off when his father waxed lyrical about her. There might have been some jealousy at work on his part that she had so much of his father's attention, and now he was stuck with her.

Far from letting her know who was in

charge here, he was about to roll up his sleeves and do her heavy lifting. Apparently the 'mug' tattoo on his forehead was still visible.

'You have got to be kidding me,' he said as they approached a very compact pastel blue Volkswagen. Which, judging by the boxes visible through the rear window, was already jam-packed.

Daisy shrugged. 'It gets me from A to B. I don't usually carry passengers of extraordinary height.'

Thomas contemplated walking to the cottage, but the extra time taken to get there would only impact further on his day. The sooner they completed this task, the quicker they could actually start work.

'So I see.' The passenger seat was pushed so far forward he had to duck to get in and fold himself over until his knees were up near his chin so he could close the door. He did not miss the smirk on Dr Swift's bright red lips as they drove away.

'Do you live close by?' she asked as she drove much faster than he liked, taking the corner without even shifting down a gear.

Thomas held onto the dashboard before he ended up sitting on her knee in the driving seat. That would probably amuse her no end, at further expense to his dignity. At least the speed with which they had accelerated away from the village meant few would have seen him hunched up in her dinky car.

Thankfully, because of her driving and the short distance they had to travel, they arrived at the cottage before his knees seized up altogether.

'Home sweet home.' Daisy was out of the vehicle carrying an armful of boxes to the door of the whitewashed building before Thomas managed to extricate himself from his pretzel position.

'I don't live in the village itself. The family home is up on the hill there.' He pointed up to the grey stone mansion isolated from the rest of the community. Thomas could not help but think they should have kept it that way, then his father would never have been hurt. It was his safe haven now. Nobody else came in and only he went out. His sanctuary and sanity when it was the one place on earth he could control. Even if it came too late to help his father.

'Very imposing and it looks down on the rest of the village. I'm sure you enjoy that.' She nudged the front door open with her hip, leaving him to follow. He did not rise to the bait when she was right, though for a different reason than she thought. It was not a feeling of superiority he got from his position up on the hill, but of safety. The distance between him and everyone else was a welcome barrier. Goodness knew what Daisy was hoping to gain from her continued quips but Thomas was not going to lose his temper over it. He supposed this life was different to the one she knew in the city. Hopefully she would either get used to it or decide it was not for her and move on quickly. Thomas knew which option he would prefer.

Although he and his father had shared the patients between them, when he had decided to retire, Thomas had tried to convince him he could manage on his own. Generations of Ryans had always staffed the local clinic and Thomas did not need a stranger moving in on his territory now. Work was all he had in his life and he needed to stay as busy as possible so he did not have time to dwell on mistakes and regret.

'I think this will do nicely.' Once she had set her boxes down, Daisy stood back to take a look around the property.

'I'm sure it's not what you're used to in London.' There wasn't a lot of space in these old places but the Ryans had always done their best to maintain the authentic feel of the village. All owned by the family, which now only consisted of himself, none of the listed buildings were for sale; they were rented by the inhabitants. At least that was one way he could keep track of who was staying. If they had allowed the cottages to be used as second homes for holidaymakers, the heart would have gone out of Little Morton a long time ago.

'No, but that's not a bad thing. At least I have more than two rooms and, bonus, no noisy neighbours on either side. Not to mention the lovely wild garden. This would cost an arm and a leg in central London and would never be half as cosy.' She plopped down on the floral sofa which came as part of the furnishings and fittings. The twee country cottage décor did not suit her. Dr Daisy Swift was a sophisticated, glamorous woman who would only ever be at home in a cityscape, he was sure.

Her white-blonde curls, piercing blue eyes and pale skin were striking. The corporate black skirt, tailored grey silk blouse and impossibly high stilettos would never fit in here, but she would find that out for herself after a few ankle-breaking days on the cobbles.

Thomas dumped his share of her belongings on the floor, sending a dust cloud up into the air, making him sneeze.

'Sorry, I think I brought that with me. A souvenir from London. These boxes haven't been unpacked since my last move. House-keeping isn't really my thing any more.' She wore a look of pride on her face as though it was a badge of honour to be so busy there was no time for something as mundane as cleaning. Yet her voice suggested something else. A past which kept her on the move.

All the more reason to be wary of her. He should have paid more attention and asked more questions about this woman who had become a big part of his father's life. As far as Daniel Ryan had been concerned, Daisy's character and qualifications were all the veri-fication needed to hire her. That was his fa-ther all over—too trusting for his own good. They had both learned that the hard way, too late. Eunice had at least suggested an inter-view, which had taken place on the internet to keep things above board. Although his fa-ther had pulled rank and insisted on conduct-ing it on his own, waiting until Thomas was away at a conference to arrange it, to ensure he could not interfere. Making her appoint-ment a foregone conclusion, no matter what Thomas had to say on the matter.

This woman had certainly had a hold on his father that unnerved him and made him suspicious about the nature of their relationship.

'If you're finished, could we get back to work please?' He was already more involved in her personal life than he wanted to be, by helping her move in when things between them should be kept strictly professional. That way he was not likely to compromise himself outside of the workplace, as he had done with Jade. What Daisy did away from the clinic had nothing to do with him and vice versa.

'There are just a few more bits and pieces. Oh, and my shoes.'

They had both traipsed out to the car where she had begun to load him up with more boxes. She had black bin bags in both hands and under her arms, which he presumed contained her now wrinkled clothes.

'Can you manage a pair of shoes?' She dangled a pair of strappy silver sandals from his finger before he could protest. His humiliation was complete when she hooked a handbag over his shoulder too.

Thomas was definitely going to have his work cut out for him, getting Dr Swift to toe the line.

* * *

'What do you do around here for fun?' Daisy cradled her well-earned cup of tea in her hands as she leaned against Thomas's desk.

The day's surgery was over at last, having run well past their official surgery hours. Judging by the minor nature of most of her patients' ailments, a lot of them had simply wanted a glimpse of the new GP. She had no idea what the verdict was, but she had felt like a mannequin in a shop window with everyone gawping at her. Only time would tell if the novelty would wear off and she would ever be considered anything other than an outsider. If she wanted to be part of the community, and she did, she would have to embrace everything they had to offer here.

It was a completely different way of life compared to the city, where she had been able to live anonymously, but she welcomed the change. She could not hide away for ever behind her workload. It meant people like her ex were still controlling her, preventing her from living her life freely and without fear.

Romantic relationships were not something she formed easily, given her lack of trust and fierce need for independence, but it shouldn't mean she couldn't have friends and neighbours to socialise with. She had forgotten that somewhere along the way, shutting everyone out, letting no one closer than on the periphery of her life. It was time to be part of something, belong somewhere, instead of merely existing.

Until now, the only people she had had a conversation with were Eunice and Thomas. Unfortunately, the friendly face around here had rushed off to babysit her grandchildren, leaving only the hard-working doctor to answer her questions. If only sighing and refusing to look up from his computer screen could be counted as a sign he was willing to accept her company.

At least he had shown her earlier he was not completely unbearable, by helping her move into the cottage. She'd had a little fun at his expense and, though his expression was priceless at having to carry her handbag and shoes, he had done so without a tantrum. There was hope he was not the stuck-up so-and-so he had projected himself as so far.

It was a shame when he was such a beautiful-looking man with his grey-blue eyes and dark blond hair. Not that Daisy was searching for a man and even if she was it would not be another one who thought he could boss her around. At least she had made it clear that was never going to happen.

'Fun?' Eventually he glanced up at her, his forehead creased into a frown.

Daisy sighed. Removing the stick from his backside was going to be harder than she'd thought. 'Yeah. Fun. The thing you do outside of work.'

'I don't really do anything.'

That didn't surprise her. He probably polished the family silver or counted his millions when he wasn't here. 'What do people do around here to socialise?'

He had to think about it. 'There's the pub or the coffee shop. We have a few festivals during the year where everyone gets together.'

Now they were getting somewhere. Daisy would be content exploring the countryside or enjoying a cup of tea in the café, but she knew she had to find some way of integrating into the village if she was to be accepted.

She wondered if their quaint festivals were like the ones she had seen on TV. Where the whole village came out to support each other, having fun at the coconut shy and kissing booths. Thomas would make a fortune if he volunteered those soft lips of his for a pound a smooch.

She sniggered, imagining some of the old dears she'd had in this morning emptying their purses for some quality time with 'that lovely Dr Ryan'.

'That sounds more like it. Do I need a pass to get into that too?' It was a tongue-in-cheek comment, but Thomas didn't appear to get the joke.

'No. Everyone is welcome to attend.'

Even you, she was sure he was silently adding.

'We have the Crab Festival next week, if you want to go to that.'

'Of course. How could I turn down a personal invitation from the Earl himself? I'd love to attend the Little Morton Crab Festival with you. I'd be honoured.'

'But that's not—'

'Thank you for making me feel so welcome on my first day, Thomas.' Daisy gave him her biggest smile and succeeded in making him shift uncomfortably in his chair.

He sighed and appeared to resign himself to the fact she was staying.

'I'm sure you will be an asset to the clinic,' he said through clenched teeth.

Once she made sure Dr Ryan knew she was no pushover, her life in Little Morton could be just the place for her to start living.

CHAPTER TWO

THOMAS HAD NO idea how he had been roped into this. Wait…yes, he did. Daisy. She had the knack of getting her own way without giving anyone the chance to say no to her. He'd also felt guilty about how he had treated her on her arrival and was now trying to build some bridges. Okay, he had his suspicions about her motives in coming here, but his father would have berated him for the way he had spoken to her on her first day. Eunice had also reminded him that they had to work together, and she had done nothing except take up the post which his father had given her. Since then, Thomas had done his best to be civil at least.

Now, not only was he down at the harbour with the rest of the village at a festival he had no interest in, but he was also sitting on a ducking stool about to be dropped into ice-cold water.

'It's for charity,' Daisy had coaxed when they had arrived and found the dunk tank was short of volunteers. He was not entirely convinced by her altruistic display, and with good reason.

'They're raising money for the lifeboat station. I'd do it myself but I'm not sure I'd get many takers.' Thomas was sure he had seen a rare flicker of fear in her eyes at the prospect, which she'd quickly blinked away, taking his arm and steering him towards the crew manning the station.

Although he would have paid good money to drop her into the tank he was currently staring down into, he could tell it was not something she would have been comfortable doing herself. The usually confident Daisy clearly had found her kryptonite and it would not have been chivalrous of him to expect her to be dunked underwater in the name of charity.

Even if she had turned his life upside down in the space of a week. Not only was she making her presence known at work, walking into his office and using his desk as a seat when drinking her countless cups of tea, but she was sneaking her way into his personal life too. He didn't usually come to these things; they were more for tourists and kids. As she was part of his medical practice he had felt obliged to help introduce her into the community so she would become familiar to the patients. His father would have wanted him to make the effort. That was uppermost in his mind when she was driving him to distraction. Thomas had to respect his father's wishes. He just didn't have to like it.

Another ball hit the canvas target beside him, completely missing the bull's-eye. So far only a few children had stepped up but he knew, come the afternoon when the dads had the chance to sample the homemade cider on Billy Jackson's stall, things could change.

With his bare feet dangling in the water and his trousers rolled up to his knees, Thomas was simply waiting for the inevitable. Especially when Daisy moved to the top of the queue, casually tossing one of the red rubber balls in her hand.

'I hope you've made your donation first, Dr Swift,' he shouted from the cage housing him and the tank of water.

Daisy waggled a ten-pound note before handing it over to the member of the lifeboat crew holding a charity box. 'I'm sure this will be worth every penny.'

She took a step back and launched the ball with more force than one would have expected from her small frame. Thomas let out a long breath as the ball smacked loudly just to the right of the target.

'So close,' he teased, and immediately regretted it when he saw the look of determination on her face as her bright red lips tightened into a thin line.

'Just getting my bearings.' She closed one eye and took aim with as much force as her first attempt. He was regretting treating her so harshly a lot right now.

Thomas barely had enough time to register the 'ding' as she hit her target before he was dropped unceremoniously into the tank. The cold water stole the oxygen from his lungs so he was gasping for air when he stood up again. He wiped his eyes and shook his head like a wet dog trying to dislodge the water from his ears. This was not the image he usually projected to the community and he couldn't say he was loving it. However, it would not have been very charitable if he'd declined to help.

'Good shot,' he spluttered as she came to high-five him, enjoying this way too much.

Thomas caught her blue eyes sweeping over his body, where his clothes were sticking to his skin, and it was then he realised he did not have a change of clothes.

* * *

Daisy had been having fun with Thomas at the dunk tank. Until now. She could not tear her eyes away from the sodden clothes clinging to his body. The wet fabric of his white shirt had turned transparent, giving her an eyeful of his muscular torso and flat stomach. Even his trousers were moulded around those thigh muscles and everything else south.

The joke had definitely backfired when she was the one who had been left blushing Although she had volunteered Thomas as one of the 'dunkees' today, it had not been a plot to humiliate him. When she had been approached to take part she had panicked at the thought of being dropped into the water. Instead, she had pushed Thomas forward to detract from any idea she should take part.

To his credit, he had agreed and saved her from making a spectacle of herself. Since their first terse exchange he had seemed to mellow a little towards her, though that could possibly have been at Eunice's urging. She had insisted Daisy had caught him on a bad day and he was not usually as abrasive as he had been with her. In fact, if Eunice was to be believed, Thomas Ryan was an absolute sweetheart of the highest order. The woman was apparently prepared to lie to make the atmosphere in the clinic more harmonious.

Daisy did get the impression he needed to integrate here as much as she did. He seemed to go between home and work with very little interaction with anyone in between. With his father gone too, he must be lonely up in that house on the hill and she knew from experience that was not fun. It was the whole reason she had moved here, to get out of that rut herself. She might not have anyone controlling her, but she was not fully living when she was afraid to let anyone get close in case she got hurt.

It was not her intention to manipulate Thomas into doing what she wanted or what she thought he needed; she would never do that to another person. He had surprised her by agreeing to accompany her here and helping out at the dunk tank. By spending the day together and seeing this co-operative side of him, it would help dispel any preconceived ideas they had of each other. She could put today down as a bonding exercise, nothing else. Certainly not an excuse to ogle her handsome work colleague.

'You're all wet,' she managed to mumble.

'I thought that was the intention when you threw the ball?' He ruffled his wet hair with his hand, making it look as though he'd just stepped out of the shower fully clothed.

Her imagination began to run rampant. Clearly her life of singledom was missing something as base as sex or she would not be fantasising about a man with whom she had absolutely nothing in common except work.

'Well, I've had my fun. I suppose I should get you a towel to dry off.'

'I'm sure I'm going to get much wetter as the day goes on. You're not the only one who apparently wants to drop me into a tank of water.' He nodded over at the queue of villagers which had formed, likely attracted by the cheering which had sounded when Daisy had dunked him in the water.

She didn't think the rush to dunk Thomas was malicious, more a novelty to see the Earl participating in such an event. To his credit, Thomas was still smiling as he climbed back onto the stool. Daisy didn't think it would do her any favours to stick around and watch the scene on repeat, or she would end up being the one who needed dunking in some cold water.

'I could take a run up to your house if you'd like and get you some dry clothes.' It was the least she could do when it was her fault he was in this predicament.

'No.' His response was short and sharp, as if the idea was completely out of the question.

'Really, it's no bother. If you give me your keys I can drive up and be back in ten minutes.'

'I said no. I'm not in the habit of letting people wander around my property unsupervised.' The gruff, unyielding doctor she had encountered on her first day was back, treating her as though she was about to single-handedly destroy life in the village as he knew it. All because she had offered to do him a favour.

Was it really so unheard of for someone to help him or did he merely have a problem accepting it from her? She wondered if she would ever know what went on in his head when he was so changeable around her. It would become exhausting trying to figure him out and Daisy hadn't moved across the country to have another man cause her stress.

'I'm not about to steal the family silver, if that's what you're worried about.' It was a throwaway comment to highlight the absurdity of his behaviour. Except the guilty look on his face told her she had hit the nail right on the head.

'It's nothing personal,' he added, only adding more heat to the burn.

'How can it be anything but personal?' She was trying not to get too animated and draw the attention of the people milling around; as a result she hissed out the words like an angry cat.

'I just don't want anyone snooping around my house.' He shrugged, unperturbed by accusing his co-worker of intending to steal from him.

Daisy had been accused of being many things over the years, but a thief was a new and unwarranted descriptor. If that was how he saw her—someone who would take advantage of him like that without her conscience pricking her—he didn't know her at all. Worse, it showed a major lack of trust and respect from someone she was supposed to be working alongside. Eunice would have to go a long way to convince her now he was a nice guy at heart and not some uppity toff who thought everyone was out to get him. She wondered who had hurt him in the past to cause this level of paranoia.

'Fine. Freeze to death. I was only trying to help, not casing the joint.' She flounced off, so angry with him that she was ready to spend the rest of the afternoon dropping him into that cold water. Her sole consolation was hearing a splash behind her as someone else did the job for her. She made her way around the rest of the fair with a smug smile.

The whole harbour was lined with stalls, colourful bunting hung from the streetlights and the noise of laughter was a glorious sound on the hot summer day. It was essentially a street party, a real community coming together for the day to have fun. There were tourists of course, keen to spend their money to join in, but Daisy recognised the majority of faces around her now.

Those who were not her patients worked in or frequented the local coffee shop and pubs, others she knew in passing. The layout of the village meant it was easy to get around on foot and there were some beautiful scenic views to be had during these promenades. She had yet to have a walk without exchanging pleasantries with others taking a stroll. So far she had not encountered any real opposition to her presence at the clinic but she did sense wariness. Especially from Thomas.

It would take time, she supposed, but she had hoped today would have gone some way towards her and Thomas bonding, as well as making their presence known more around the village. Now she felt more unwanted than ever.

'Hi, Dr Swift. Would you care to try some

of our homemade fudge?' The woman behind the sweet stall was one of Daisy's new patients, Marie Talbot. She had brought a basket of chocolate chip muffins in on Daisy's first day, so she would always be one of her favourite people. Today her warm smile and sugary treats were especially welcomed.

'I would love some, Marie. Thank you.' Daisy took one of the small samples laid out for potential customers to taste and let the sugary sweetness dissolve on her tongue.

'What's the verdict?' The pretty mum of two waited for her review even though she had other customers lining up.

'I think my waistline is in trouble.' She handed over her money in exchange for the bag of fudge tied with curled pink ribbon which she would comfort eat later when she replayed her conversation with Thomas alone in the cottage.

By the time she circled back to the dunk tank, Thomas, having finished his stint as a merman, was there waiting for her. He had changed into dry clothes which someone had apparently donated. The tight white T-shirt with *Little Morton Crab Festival* emblazoned in bright pink and colourful board shorts were not quite his style but still managed to catch her attention.

Daisy was trying not to stare at the water dripping from his hair down the front of his shirt or the drops sitting on the ends of his long eyelashes like early morning dew on the grass when she was still mad at him.

'I'll see you on Monday at work,' she said, turning away, having seen and heard enough of him for more than one day.

'Wait. I'm sorry about what I said earlier. I've had plenty of time to think it over in between dunkings. I didn't mean to offend you. I just don't let anyone into my house.'

'No one?' Daisy was not a party girl who invited all and sundry back to her house, and she understood the need for privacy, but Thomas's attitude was a tad over-the-top in her opinion.

'No one. So you see—it's not you, it's me.' The big warm smile he sent her was equally unsettling, as though she had watched him change right in front of her. It was Thomas, naked, no longer hiding behind that stern façade she had first encountered.

'Uh huh. Well, perhaps you should remember that next time you're about to snap at me.' She should have dug deeper to find out the reason behind his fierce protection of his personal space, but she might regret chipping away at that hard exterior when Thomas's soft inner core was even more terrifying. She didn't want to like him, given his propensity to make her feel small, no matter how unintentionally. It was important she started expanding her social pool here so Thomas Ryan wasn't the only person in the village she was getting to know on a personal level.

'Sorry. I'm not used to sharing any aspect of my personal space since my father died. I will do my best to think before I speak in future. Can I buy you some lunch by way of apology?'

'I suppose so.' Although she should let him sweat a bit longer, it wouldn't help their situation by refusing his olive branch or, in this case, the smell of salt and vinegar emanating from the catering vans.

They ordered some fish and chips to share and sat down on the harbour wall to eat it.

Thomas plonked the bag containing his wet clothes on the ground and helped himself to some of the golden chips fresh out of the fryer. 'I'm starving.'

'How come you don't usually go to these things? It's been fun today and I think everyone is glad to see you.'

He shrugged his shoulders. 'I used to come when I was little but school and work soon took up most of my time. I don't know… I suppose I thought it could diminish my reputation here. My father was a well-respected man and I felt the pressure to be like him. I'm doing my best to honour him wherever I can.'

'Is that why you don't want me working at the clinic with you?'

He blinked, the chip he was holding hovering on its way to his mouth. 'That's not—'

'There's no need to deny it. I think it was obvious to me and poor Eunice that you weren't happy about my arrival from day one.'

Thomas hung his head before glancing up at her from below those lovely long lashes. 'I apologise if I didn't make you feel welcome. I've been wary of outsiders since my father's death and, well, I don't know anything about you beyond your CV. He was the one who hired you, who considered you a friend, but you're a stranger to me. You could have been coming out here to stake a claim on his money for all I knew.'

There was so much information there to make Daisy uncomfortable, but it was just the truth and she should be thankful for that at least.

However, he was still talking about her as though she was a threat to him, when she'd thought they'd been making progress up until today. He didn't say he'd changed his opinion about her or that he realised she was not here because she was interested in his father's money and that was difficult to accept. She would have to double her efforts for him to appreciate she was good at her job and work was the only reason she was here.

'Why would your father's death affect your trust in people who come from outside the village? I don't understand.' If she did, it might go some way to explaining his attitude towards her.

Thomas launched his chip into the sea for the hungry seagulls to dive upon, his appetite apparently deserting him as she touched on the subject of his father's passing.

Obviously his grief was raw, when Dr Ryan senior had died only months ago, but Daisy suspected there was more going on here than mourning.

'As you know, he was a great believer in helping others and was involved in a number of good causes.'

Daisy nodded. If it hadn't been for the Earl's scholarship programme she would never have escaped that prison her ex had kept her in through sheer fear alone.

'He was a very generous man. I owe him a lot.'

Thomas huffed out a breath, suggesting he wasn't in complete agreement with some of his father's practices.

'What does that mean?' Her hackles were rising now at the suggestion that she might have been taking advantage of his father's kind nature in some way.

Although the scholarship had been arranged through a third party, Daisy had written to the Earl to express her gratitude and explain what it meant to her. Freedom. She liked to think they had struck up a real friendship, keeping in touch about her progression through medical school and beyond. The Earl, in turn, had told her about village life, sufficient to make her fall in love with the place without ever having seen it. In his letters he had told of his pride in his son and she'd hoped he'd passed on some kind words about her to his heir. However, it seemed Thomas thought of her as no more than a gold-digger. That hurt. Part of the reason she had come here was to repay the Earl's kindness by filling in the gap in his medical practice, but she got the impression Thomas saw her as someone who had wormed her way into his father's affections and his wallet. Now her motives for being here were in question it tainted the new start she had hoped to have here.

Once more she was forced to justify her presence here, but she wouldn't do it at any cost. If they couldn't get past their differences she would have to move on. She was not going to spend any more of her life believing she wasn't worthy of her place.

'It means he thought with his heart instead of his head and acted accordingly.'

Something Thomas would never be accused of doing.

Before Daisy drew herself up to her full height with the offence she had taken at that comment, Thomas carried on with his explanation.

'He trusted too easily and apparently so did I.'

She snorted at that, but he ignored her derision.

'When I was away at a medical conference, some people broke into the house. They tied him up and beat him before stealing whatever they could find.' Thomas picked some small stones up from the ground and fired them into the water one by one. Perhaps in an attempt to rid himself of all the things which were bothering him.

'I'm sorry you both had to deal with that. Your father was such a lovely, generous man. He did not deserve that.' Daisy's stomach lurched violently at the thought of the Earl being subjected to such brutality when he had been kindness personified. It was understandable that Thomas should be bitter about what had happened, but she was having trouble putting the pieces together. 'Forgive me for saying, but I thought your father died from heart failure?'

As the date for her start date had grown near and she hadn't heard from the Earl, Daisy had phoned the clinic. That was when Eunice had broken the news to her that he had passed away in hospital. There hadn't been any mention of a robbery or an assault. It would have compounded her grief, as it apparently had with Thomas. Gradually, she was beginning to see why Thomas acted the way he did around her.

'Ultimately, that's what killed him, but his health took a sharp decline after the incident. In the year after it happened he became very stressed about his personal security, to the point of paranoia. Understandably so, but I don't think he ever felt safe again in his own home. That was down to me. I should have been there to protect him.'

'I can see why you would feel that way, but the only people to blame are those who carried out that heinous act.' She could only imagine the Earl's terror and Thomas's shock when he had heard what had happened to his father in his absence. It would have been traumatic for both of them.

Even now, picturing the horrific scene herself made her want to weep for the sweet man who had given her a second chance at life. The Earl had only deserved good things to happen to him and hearing what he had gone through, how he had suffered as a result, was devastating. She had come to Little Morton partly to try and repay his kindness, but she would never get to do that because of the evil act of greedy, unscrupulous people. He hadn't told her about the robbery but she suspected his pride had prevented him from sharing the traumatic events with her. Another layer of sadness was added to her loss that she never had the opportunity to comfort the man who had done so much for her. It would have destroyed the Earl to realise they had gone to his home with no compunction about hurting him when he'd only ever done good. Daisy would have found it equally as hard as Thomas to forgive or trust again.

'They were caught, judged and given pitiful sentences for their act. It gives me no comfort to know they're in jail. Their incarceration makes no difference. It won't bring my father back.'

It was easy to see how a grieving son would blame himself for his father's untimely death and it explained why he had been so against the idea of a stranger joining the practice or being in his home. If they had exercised that same caution before now, perhaps the Earl would not have suffered as much as he had.

Although Thomas seemed to be getting used to her, Daisy was certain trust wasn't something he would give easily again. That was something they had in common. Her experiences in the past meant she was always waiting for people to reveal a darker side. Like her stepfamily and her ex. Unfortunately she was usually proved right in her need to be cautious. When people didn't get what they wanted their true colours would appear, warning her to back away.

These days she didn't hang around when someone proved untrustworthy. It could be that Thomas was waiting for her to slip up too and give him a reason to get rid of her in case someone else got hurt. It was lucky for both of them that she had no hidden agenda. She was honest and forthright and appreciated people who were the same. As long as they didn't try to tell her what to do or how to behave…

'Anyway, I should get going. I think I've done enough socialising for one day.' Just like that, Thomas ended their lunch and the conversation, apparently coming to the conclusion that they should keep their relationship strictly professional and within the walls of the clinic too.

There was nothing Daisy could say or do to change his mind over the burden of guilt he was carrying, but hopefully he would see she had no ulterior motive in moving out to Little Morton other than to start her life anew. She would prove to him that his father had known best by bringing her here, simply by doing her job.

CHAPTER THREE

COME MONDAY MORNING, Daisy was on board with the idea that her relationship with Thomas should be strictly professional. She had no right to know the ins and outs of his personal life and vice versa. It would keep things simpler. As long as he could do the same and remember she was here as a GP and not some con woman who had come to squeeze money out of him now his father had gone.

She still respected his position as the senior partner and when she wanted a second opinion concerning one of her patients she didn't think twice about seeking his opinion.

'I'm going to go and talk to my colleague for a moment. It's nothing to worry about. I just want to consult him on this,' she told her young patient as she left the room. He had presented to her with an itchy red rash on and around his thighs. Normally she would have put it down to prickly heat or an allergy but the intense itching he was describing, along with a recent trip to Florida, made her think it might be something else, especially when she did some quick online research into the area where he had been staying.

The door to Thomas's room was slightly ajar but she knocked out of courtesy and waited for a response.

'Yes?'

'Sorry to disturb you, Thomas, but I was wondering if I could get a second pair of eyes on a patient next door.'

'Sure. What's up?' He set down the pen he had been writing with and gave her his complete attention.

'I have a young surfer in his twenties who has just returned from Florida. He has a red bumpy rash in his groin/inner thigh area which is causing him severe itching. Something tells me it's not the usual summer allergies we're dealing with here. I've found there's something called Seabather's Eruption which can occur and wondered if you had ever come across this before.'

Thomas got up from behind the desk, ready to see the patient's predicament for himself. 'Is he experiencing any vomiting, headaches or fatigue?'

'Not so far. It's the itching which is mainly

bothering him, apart from the unsightliness of the rash, of course.'

'I'll take a look,' he said, following her back into her own room.

'Thanks.' Although Daisy could happily have prescribed treatment which would cover most allergic reactions or skin rashes, she preferred to find out exactly what she was dealing with for future reference. If that meant asking someone with more experience for his opinion, so be it. The patient was more important than her pride.

'Hi, I'm Dr Ryan. Dr Swift tells me you have come home from Florida with a nasty rash. Would you mind if I took a look?' Thomas washed his hands before pulling back the curtain around the bed in the corner.

Justin the surfer joined him in the cubicle for the consultation while Daisy waited.

'I think you're right, Dr Swift. It's not something we would commonly deal with in the UK, but I have seen this before when I did a placement in dermatology. A chap came back from his honeymoon in Mexico with the same unfortunate problem.' Thomas washed and dried his hands again as Justin emerged from behind the curtain.

'Is it serious?'

'Not at all. There are a lot of names for it—Seabather's Eruption, pica-pica, marine dermatitis—but it's all the same thing. Basically, it's caused by stings from certain sea anemones or thimble jellyfish. The rash is concentrated on your bottom half as it's believed the tiny organisms get trapped under the bathing suit, against the skin there.'

Justin turned up his nose at the thought. 'Does that mean these things are still living on me?'

'No. This is simply an allergic response to the stings. Just make sure you thoroughly wash whatever you were wearing in the water at the time. Dr Swift will prescribe you some steroids and some antihistamines to reduce the severity of the itching. If you experience any other symptoms such as a fever or nausea, do come back and see us.' Thomas made his way out of the room and Daisy offered her thanks as she saw him out.

'Good call. Not many would have gone the extra mile to look into that beyond the initial symptoms.' Thomas's praise warmed her and she hoped he was beginning to see she took her job and her patients seriously. It would make things easier for her here, as well as improving relations between them.

* * *

'What a day.' Daisy bumped open the door into Thomas's office with her hip and walked in carrying two mugs of tea.

'What's this in aid of?' he asked a little suspiciously. At the start of the day she'd seemed distant with him and he'd wondered if he had upset her at the festival with his honesty. Normally he wouldn't have given away so much personal information, but he thought he owed her some explanation for the way he'd behaved towards her. When he'd realised he had perhaps overshared, he had tried to put some distance between them. It seemed to have stuck but at least Daisy had felt able to come to him earlier about her patient. Hopefully he hadn't ruined the rapport they had managed to build and they'd be able to work together as a team here at the clinic.

'I thought it would be good for us to debrief at the end of the day. You know, talk over our cases, see if there is anything that warrants both our attention. The best way to do that is over a cup of tea.' She set a cup in front of him, then slid his files to one side so she could lean back against his desk.

'Generally, we do that during our morning staff meetings.' In the company of their other colleagues and in the staffroom.

'I know, but I thought we could start our own routine with things still fresh in our minds. It will give us a chance to catch up and swap notes.' Daisy kicked off her heels so she was barefoot as she lounged against the desk.

'There is another seat, you know.' He indicated the empty seat next to her. There was something unnerving about having her hover in his office, making herself at home like this. Even though this was within the boundaries of their professional relationship, it still felt intimate, too familiar for his liking.

'I've spent most of the day sitting down. I want to stretch my legs,' she said, ignoring his discomfort.

'So…is there anything you need to urgently discuss about today's patients?' If she insisted on doing this then he wanted to get it over with as quickly as possible and send her on her way.

'The only thing that really stands out is our surfer with the rash, Justin. That's one I will have to remember in case I come across anything like it again.' She seemed pleased to have discovered the cause of the young patient's problem and rightly so. It wasn't every day that they successfully diagnosed a tropical illness without the intervention of a specialist. That was down to her determination to diagnose on sight. It was lucky that he had seen that particular rash before to confirm her suspicions, so it had been a successful collaboration he hoped they would see more of together.

'That was well spotted. I was impressed.'

'Not as much as I was to learn you had treated the condition before. Remind me to come to you for all the rare and unusual cases which come through the door.' She was teasing him, but Thomas appreciated the respect she was showing him and his experience rather than insisting she knew best in all cases. It was better for their patients to have two doctors who worked well together to provide the best treatment for all.

'We're on the coast so we get a lot of surfers and divers. It's only to be expected that we'll get the odd rarity from someone who has taken their hobby abroad. It's not just all hip replacements and hearing aids in Little Morton, you know.' He couldn't resist a little joke of his own and it was nice to know there were still some surprises to be had in their sleepy village. It might prevent the city girl from getting bored and seeking some excitement outside the clinic.

'Do you need a lift home? The rain is pouring down out there.' Thomas poked his head around Daisy's office door.

'No, thanks. I've a lot of paperwork to catch up on here.' Her fingers were flying over the keyboard much quicker than he had ever managed. Although it wouldn't surprise him if she was simply pretending to have a heavy workload so they didn't break their unspoken 'no fraternising away from work' rule.

Thomas hoped he hadn't offended her by talking about his distrust of 'outsiders' after the festival. Whilst he didn't know a lot about her background, she was fitting in well with everyone at the clinic after her first couple of weeks. It would be a while before he could fully trust her, if ever, but he had to think about the welfare of their patients and Daisy was a good doctor. He no longer had the urge to run her out of town. If anything, it was the opposite. They worked well as a team here and she was fun to be around.

It was probably for the best that they didn't spend their personal time together. Seeing each other too much could be a bad thing when they were together all day at work too. Over-familiarity could turn out to be detrimental when he had so much going on. Not only was he the lead in the clinic but he'd had to take on his father's other projects too. He didn't have time for anyone, or anything, else.

However, he'd got used to her popping into his office uninvited for a chat or bringing him a cup of tea every time she made herself one. That was one of her quirks. He had never seen someone drink so much tea and he had added a decaf option in the staffroom for the sake of her health, and his. So far, she had not seemed to avail herself of the alternative.

Now Daisy was here he no longer had to deal with everything on his own. He had been prepared to do that on a work basis when his father had talked of retiring, but Thomas had not expected to lose him altogether. Without his presence at home or work, life had become *too* quiet. At least with Daisy he had someone to talk to about patients or the day he'd had.

'I can wait. I'll make us a cuppa and hopefully the rain will have died down by then.' He headed off to the staffroom without giving her the chance to refuse again.

There was no way he was going to let her walk home in torrential rain simply to avoid spending time with him outside of work. They could make an exception in this sort of circumstance.

It was a while before she conceded and finally left her office with her coat and bag in hand. Thomas would have been willing to sit it out all night if he'd had to. It was not as though he had anyone waiting at home for him.

'I'm ready to go,' she said on her way to wash her cup in the sink.

Thomas would have been in danger of dozing off in the armchair waiting for her if it had not been for the rain thudding on the roof and pelting against the staffroom windows.

'Then what are we waiting for?' He bounced up out of the chair with more enthusiasm than was called for, but he wanted her to know he was happy to give her a lift.

She walked most days but, as he lived further away and had his own parking space, Thomas usually drove to work. It wouldn't have been very chivalrous of him to leave her to walk home in this weather while he stayed warm and dry in his car.

It was so overcast outside when they did leave the clinic he wondered if he had fallen asleep after all and had slept half the night away. The wind was whipping up a frenzy, with bits of branches and other debris spiralling up into the sky. However, it was the amount of rain which had apparently fallen which was causing him most concern.

The drains were bubbling up and there was

a deluge of water running down the length and breadth of the main street.

'I think we should check on the river out by your place, just in case there is a danger of it bursting its banks.' He didn't want to worry her unnecessarily but the cottage was the closest building and there was a chance that it could be in danger. Historically, there had been one or two incidents of flooding from the river, but not for a long time. There had been some rain forecast but not to this extent or they would have taken precautions earlier.

As the owner, any damage would have to be repaired by him, so it was in his best interest to prevent it if possible. Okay, he was concerned about Daisy's safety too. With the boundaries they appeared to have created, he couldn't be certain she would come to him if she needed any help.

'I'm sure it will be fine. Isn't the river under your jurisdiction too? I doubt it would risk your wrath by going against any of your rules.' Although he could see her slight grin in his rear-view mirror, he wondered if the distance between them was about more than maintaining a professional relationship. Perhaps she had a problem with the fact he pretty much ran the village. He didn't want to use the word

'dictated' but Daisy might if she was too sti-
fled by the way things worked around here.
Thomas wanted her to feel comfortable, part
of the community, but for his father's sake
and everyone else in Little Morton he had to
be careful.

'Well, if it hasn't got a pass, it's not getting
in.' He attempted some humour but as they
pulled up outside the cottage the joke was
forgotten when they saw how dangerous the
situation outside was becoming.

Even in the early evening gloom the flooded
fields surrounding the house were apparent,
the water obliterating everything but the highest ground. Thankfully, the cottage was not
submerged, but that could be just a matter of
time. Sitting away from the main street, it was
hidden from view or one of the other residents
would have noticed and forewarned them.

They stepped out of the car and found
themselves ankle-deep in water. He saw the
wide-eyed look of panic on Daisy's face.

'How are we going to stop it getting into
the house?'

Despite the gravity of the situation and the
costly implications for him, Thomas was glad
she was including him in resolving this problem with her. The way things had been, she
might have insisted she could deal with ev-

erything herself. It left an opening for him to do something, hopefully without being accused of being too domineering.

'There are some sandbags out in the shed. We can stack those up against the doors and keep our fingers crossed that does the job. I'll phone the council and the water company and anyone else who can come and help.' He let Daisy lead the way to one of the outbuildings behind the house. She didn't hesitate in shifting the heavy sandbags, unperturbed by her ruined shoes or waterlogged trousers.

Thomas continued to be impressed by her work ethic, even though he had seen it in abundance at the clinic. Patients loved her sympathetic nature, along with that same determination he could see now as she got to the root of people's ailments and sought suitable treatment. She was certainly earning her place and he silently thanked his father for knowing best in this instance. If Thomas had been forced to fill the vacancy at the practice he would have wanted a local replacement and could have struggled with double the workload if Daisy hadn't been so persistent in the face of his reticence.

Once Thomas had notified all the relevant authorities, emergency services and as many residents as he had in his phone book that there could be a risk of flooding, he loaded up with sandbags to shore up the back of the cottage. Although the village was experiencing the effects of the strong winds and the road was slick with rain, there was no indication down there of the possible catastrophe heading their way.

'What about the rest of the village? Should we start warning people?' Daisy, like him, was soaked through but undeterred as the wind and rain battered her. Her hair was plastered to her face, the rain dripping off her chin as she shivered with cold.

'I've phoned ahead and I'm going there next. If you're coming, put something warm and dry on. I don't suppose you've got a pair of wellies?'

She took time to give him a dirty look. 'You've seen my shoe collection.'

'Not to worry. I think I have some in the boot of my car. I'll finish here; you go and get changed.'

'What about you? You're soaked too.'

'I'll manage. I'm going to get a whole lot wetter soon anyway. You don't have to come if you want to stay and get your things out of harm's way. Just in case.'

She didn't take time to consider it. 'No. I want to help.'

'Okay then, go and get changed. You'll be no use to me with pneumonia.' He shooed her away and carried on heaving the sand-bags between the buildings until he had utilised all of them.

Thomas hoped for Daisy's sake they did the job they were supposed to do when she didn't have a lot of belongings she could afford to lose, never mind her home.

As soon as she appeared again in suitable layers of warm clothing and a waterproof jacket, they jumped into the car. Other than to continue warning people of the potential flood risk, he didn't know what else they could do but they would damn well try to prevent a tragedy befalling the village. It would be his worst fear come true to see the place destroyed with no way of him preventing it. For the second time in his life he felt completely powerless.

Daisy's heart was in her throat as they drove towards the village. Thomas's forehead was almost touching the windscreen trying to see where he was going. The rain was coming so fast and heavy now the wipers couldn't keep up, making visibility next to impossible. Despite their impatience to get through, the conditions meant they were moving at a slower pace than either of them wanted. The roads were already treacherous, the water swirling around the car, detritus hitting the roof and blocking their path.

'I'm going to park at the top of the village at the barrier.' He didn't have to say any more. It was obvious why he wasn't risking driving any further when Daisy was worried too that they might get washed down the road and into the harbour. It didn't bear thinking about.

For one thing, she couldn't swim. Even if she had faced her fear of water to learn, that level of independence hadn't been encouraged by either her stepfather or her ex, and hobbies weren't something she'd had time for in London. If she survived this, it was something she would look into, in case near-drowning was a common occurrence in these parts.

She shuddered, but this time through fear rather than from the cold. Thanks to Thomas she was at least warm and better prepared to go back out into the storm.

A glance across at him told her his suit and shoes were ruined. Goodness knew how he or his clothes would ever dry out when he was saturated. Guilt clawed at her, knowing he had stood out in that rain working to protect her home whilst she'd had a chance to change. He had even been prepared to sacrifice his wellies for her but she had found an old pair of boots in her wardrobe which she had worn once to a festival and were more practical than heels at least.

'Don't forget your wellies,' she called to him as he got out of the car. Not that they would make much difference to him now, but he did stop at the rear of the car to retrieve them.

When Daisy stepped out she nearly lost her footing altogether, the water was rushing down past them so fast. She had to take a few deep breaths to regulate her heartbeat after the shock.

'This is bad. Are you sure you want to do this? I'd prefer to get you to safety. You could take the keys to the clinic if you want.'

She was touched by his concern, and tempted to get out of harm's way, but Thomas couldn't rouse the whole village alone.

'Don't worry. I'm made of tough stuff.' Although she was projecting a bravado she did not feel when she was so frightened of losing her footing and somehow ending up underwater, fighting to breathe, her lungs filling up...

'I never doubted that.' He smiled and took her hand as they waded down the street. Daisy knew it was only to keep them both anchored, but it was nice to feel the warm security of his large hand in hers. She kept a tight hold and not only because she needed him to keep her upright. It had been a long time since anyone had wanted to hold her hand. Longer still since she had allowed it.

'For the record, you need to know in case I get swept out to sea or something, I can't swim. I hate the water. So if you see me bobbing about in the harbour you'll have to throw me a lifebelt.' She didn't wish to feel too comfortable with him and the prospect of death by drowning was a subject guaranteed to keep her mind occupied elsewhere.

'I think I'd try harder than that to save you, Daisy. I'd be straight in there after you.' He squeezed her hand to reassure her and though she stopped believing he would let her drown, it did the opposite when it came to her growing feelings towards him and made her feel as though she was in too deep already. Thankfully, Thomas couldn't tell what was going on in her head and kept hold of her hand the rest of the way down the street.

The residents Thomas had sent urgent text messages to were already out, trying to block the fronts of their houses. Nevertheless, they went door to door knocking frantically and shouting out for everyone to hear. By the time they reached the bottom of the hill there was a torrent of water carrying all sorts of debris down the main street.

'Watch out!' She tugged Thomas back as someone's garden bench came rushing down past them.

'We should wait this out indoors. I don't think there's much else we can do until the emergency services get here.' It was he who made the call to put their safety first, just as a loud roar sounded somewhere behind them.

He unlocked the shutters on the medical centre, pulling Daisy inside the door just as a tidal wave appeared to engulf the street outside. Cars, trees and anything else shaken loose by the storm were being washed away down the road.

Daisy could only watch in horror as Little Morton disappeared under water. She rested her head on Thomas's broad shoulder, knowing he must be devastated too when this was his village and his buildings being destroyed before his eyes. Even now the water was pouring in under the door and invading their refuge.

'We need to get to higher ground, but I don't want to risk going out there again. There's an old attic we use for storage if you don't mind the dark?' Thomas grabbed a long wooden pole from behind Reception and hooked a hidden hatch up in the hallway ceiling.

'I'll take it over dirty water,' she muttered as it was now swirling around her ankles.

'We can sit it out up here until it's safe to come down. There's no way of knowing how high the water levels will get. You go on up and I'll try to move as much equipment as I can out of harm's way.' He brought a stepladder down for her but there was no way she was letting him do all the hard graft on his own again.

'You know that's not going to work for me, right?'

Daisy saw a flicker of a smile on his lips as he nodded and stopped waiting for her to climb the ladder.

Between them they unplugged the electrical equipment, including the computers, and moved them and the patient files out of imminent danger. Once the water was close to waist-deep, Thomas grabbed his medical bag and insisted they made a move to safety.

From the safety of the loft they watched in despair as the water continued to rise below.

'I hope everyone else is safe,' he said, watching his own property being destroyed.

'We gave everyone as much warning as we

could. With any luck they'll all be waiting this out like us. However long that may be.' If this lasted all night they were not going to have the best night's sleep in their wet clothes on these hard floorboards lining the attic space.

Thomas had used the light on his phone to show the way since the electricity had cut out and all she could see up here were boxes of old files and Christmas decorations. Nothing that was going to provide any comfort during the storm.

'I did manage to salvage something…'

Daisy could see the glint in his eye as he reached around for something behind him. She wondered if he had a practical radio or something more personal and sentimental. When he produced a flask of tea and biscuits from his medical bag she laughed out loud.

'Tea? At a time like this?'

'Essential emergency supplies for a rural GP who might find himself stranded, miles away from the nearest kettle. Anyway, it's the best thing for shock. Tell me you're not dying for a cup.'

She could have kissed him as he poured the comforting beverage into two tin mugs and handed one to her. Instead, she let her mouth savour the chocolate biscuit she had taken from the packet.

'There's nothing we can do yet. We're best up here out of the way. Safe. I can't see the water reaching us here, but in the worst-case scenario we can get out onto the roof from here.' Thomas reminded her that if not for him she could have been washed away like one of the cars being carried down towards the harbour as though they were nothing. If he hadn't convinced her to accept a lift home she would have been caught by the storm and the flood. All because she was dodging being with him.

She took another bite of her biscuit. That plan had worked out well. Not. She had to face it, there was no escaping him when their lives were so closely entwined.

'Thank you for everything tonight. You've been very kind. Amazingly so.' When she had first arrived she would never have expected the stuck-up Dr Ryan to turn out to be the local hero. He had literally waded into the middle of this crisis in his expensive suit without a thought for himself, only for others in the village, including her. It was not in keeping with the plan to keep things strictly professional.

'It's nothing anybody else wouldn't have done.'

Daisy didn't want to like him as much as

she did right now, but damn it if he wasn't making that impossible as he shrugged off the compliment.

She finished her biscuit and washed it down with some tea and began to think about everything which had brought her to this moment.

'I broke up with someone recently; that's why I decided to move here and start again.'

Thomas set his cup down and fixed her with those incredible blue eyes. 'I ended a relationship recently too. I know I've been difficult to work with at times, but I enjoy your company. You're not afraid of hard work or telling me if you think I'm out of order.'

'You do need coaxing down out of your ivory tower sometimes. Speaking of which, what about your place? You've been so busy helping everyone else you haven't checked there for possible damage.'

'It should be okay with the house being on higher ground. There's no one there to get hurt. Not any more.' Daisy wouldn't have been human if she hadn't reached out when he was clearly still in pain over his loss. Vulnerable.

A hug was the sort of comfort people gave each other every day. Not Daisy. She held hands, consoled people who might have had bad news, but hugs were too intimate for her to casually give away. It was different with Thomas. She could sense he needed one as much as she did. This human contact, compassion and sheer need to be held.

He buried his nose in her hair. Daisy breathed in the scent of him, so reassuring during this chaos. She was grateful for his support, for not giving up on her even when she had pushed him away. Most of all, he was a reminder that she didn't have to be alone. In times like this it was comforting to have someone to lean on.

However, her relationship status was a conscious decision she had made and with good reason. Those feel-good hormones that came with a hug or a kiss didn't last long and they certainly weren't worth the long-term consequences of being stuck with another controlling man. They didn't come much more controlling than the Earl who owned the whole village. These days Daisy didn't do serious romantic entanglements and getting involved with her co-worker/boss/landlord had major flashing warning lights. She would be a fool to ignore them.

CHAPTER FOUR

'THE RAIN SOUNDS as though it's dying down.' Daisy released Thomas from her embrace and moved away to reclaim some personal space.

'Yeah, and I think the water's beginning to subside down there.'

Daisy couldn't tell if it had or if he was making an excuse to escape this sudden awkwardness between them too.

'Be careful.' She didn't want him in danger simply because they'd had a moment and were both regretting it.

'I'm just going to take a look outside.' Thomas jumped down out of the loft with a splash. He cleared the obstacles swimming in his path and gently eased the door open.

Daisy held her breath, worried another wave might suddenly sweep in and overwhelm him. Thankfully, the water swishing around him didn't rise any more than knee height, so she could breathe again.

'How does it look out there?' she shouted, keen to abandon their hiding place to explore with him.

'I think it's safe enough for you to come down.'

That was all the encouragement she needed to wade out into the street after him. The rain was easing off and though there was a river flowing down the street, the immediate danger appeared to have passed. Some of the other residents had ventured out to inspect the carnage too. Most were dressed in waterproofs and she could even see others using inflatable dinghies as their mode of transport.

'We should check everyone's okay.' Typically, he wasn't thinking of himself or his own losses first. Daisy respected him so much on a personal and professional level it made her wish even more she had met his father to thank him for his amazing son along with all of his other good work.

'I'll get some supplies in case we need them.' Daisy trudged through the clinic to retrieve her medical bag. Hopefully everyone had been given time to get to safety but, until the emergency services got through, she and Thomas would be the only medics on scene.

He was already banging on doors and talking to neighbours by the time she joined him outside. 'Is everyone inside all right?'

'I'll check the other side of the street.' Daisy left him so they could move quickly from house to house doing their welfare checks.

Most people were generally upset and in shock but without any serious injuries to report. She put that down to Thomas's quick thinking in warning them, getting everyone to safety as soon as possible.

Once they reached the bottom of the hill they met up to compare notes.

'A few people are shaken up, but all accounted for here,' he reported back.

'Pretty much the same on this side. A lot of people took refuge up in the function room at the bar. There might be a few sore heads in the morning but nothing to warrant serious concern. The only place I didn't get any answer from was the cottage on the corner. I don't think I've ever seen who lives there. Is it empty?' She had knocked on the door and the windows but had not seen any sign of life about the place.

Thomas's frown immediately rang warning bells. 'Hmm. That's old Jimmy's place. He doesn't usually go too far from the house so he should be there. I'll try him again in case he didn't hear you.'

They hot-footed it over to the cottage and Thomas hammered on the front door. 'Jimmy? It's Thomas Ryan. I want to make sure you're all right in there.'

When there was no answer Daisy peered in the window, but couldn't see anyone inside. 'He's not in the front room.'

Some more hammering and shouting followed but they received only silence in response.

'Wait. Can you hear that?' Thomas stilled, listening, on alert for any noise.

Daisy was about to tell him he must have imagined it when she thought she heard a faint voice. 'I think it's coming from around the back.'

'Jimmy likes to tinker with old cars out there.' Thomas started off around the side of the house and Daisy went after him. The place looked as though it was being used as a junkyard and it was surprising Thomas let him get away with hoarding so many unsightly car parts and engines when the rest of the village was picture postcard perfect. At least it had been, until the flood had wreaked havoc.

He must have seen her expression as they squeezed past an old washing machine jammed up against the wall beside a broken Welsh dresser. 'It seems as though he's collecting more than car parts these days. He's an old friend of the family so he gets special dispensation, but I think I'll have to have a word with him about health and safety matters.'

That went some way to explaining why this had been allowed to get so out of control, but Daisy thought it was also partly due to Thomas knowing it would make the old man happy to let him get on with it. It had become a death-trap though now the water had shifted some of the heavy white goods into precarious positions. As proved when they heard another faint cry for help coming from somewhere behind all the chaos.

'Jimmy? It's Thomas Ryan.'

Another pained sound and what she thought was splashing sent them running to find the source of the noise. The back garden was a veritable swimming pool with the old cars and stacked household appliances around the perimeter.

'Help!' A silver head was bobbing up out of the water beside one clapped-out old vehicle.

They both rushed over to give assistance in the waist-deep water. Jimmy was spluttering, clinging to the body of the car in an up-

right position, trying to keep his head above
the surface.

'My leg's stuck… I think it's broken. I
jacked the car up so I could take a look un-
derneath at the chassis but the whole thing
collapsed on me. Next thing I knew a river
of water had flooded the yard and nearly
drowned me.' The old man was clearly in pain
and gasping for air. It seemed as though he
hadn't secured the vehicle properly. Given the
state of the place, she didn't think he took his
health and safety seriously and was now suf-
fering the consequences.

'We might need the fire brigade to move
this off you, but we'll do our best, Jimmy.
Daisy, can you make sure his head stays
above water and keep him talking? I'll get
down and take a look at the leg.' Thomas
stripped off his sodden outer layer and with
one deep breath dipped below the water.
There was no thought given to the dirty water
he was immersing himself in, he was so focused on helping. They would all need to be
hosed down after this and perhaps have to
take antibiotics as a preventative measure
against any nasty bacteria lurking in there.

'It's going to be all right, Jimmy. Help is on
the way.' She was using all her body weight to
prop him up, his head leaning back against her

chest. He was tiring, his body weak. They'd got here in the nick of time. Thanks to Thomas.

Thomas had to feel around the leg to see where Jimmy was injured and how he was trapped. It was not going to be easy to get him out, and it would be painful, but it was also necessary. Not only could an open wound get infected from the dirty water, but they couldn't keep him afloat indefinitely. At the moment Jimmy was able to co-operate but if he lost consciousness or went into shock they would struggle to save him.

Thomas resurfaced to take a breath, gasping greedily for air. 'On initial examination I think we're dealing with a compound fracture to the tibia. I can feel the bone poking through the skin. I need to free the leg before we can treat it. This isn't going to be pleasant, Jimmy. Honestly, it will hurt like hell but I'll be as quick as I can.'

Ideally they would align the bones and immobilise the leg so it could heal properly but, given the situation, their priority was to get Jimmy out from under the car and out of the water. Until then, there could be all sorts of complications, such as infection setting into the open wound from the dirty water or hypothermia or shock setting in because of the cold. It was likely he was going to need surgery to align the bone properly and a cast to help stabilise it, but they could do all that at the hospital. For now, the important thing was to get him somewhere dry and keep him conscious.

'Do what you have to, Doc. I don't know how much longer I can hang on.'

'Daisy, if I can brace my weight against the car, I need you to pull the leg free.' It meant she would have to go underwater but it was the only way they could get Jimmy out.

She nodded. 'Jimmy, you'll have to support yourself until we get this done, okay?'

'Whatever it takes,' the old man replied.

'Okay then, let's do this.' Thomas was looking at Daisy as he said it, doing his best to express his support when he knew that she was not comfortable in the water.

She helped manoeuvre Jimmy so he could hold on to the car door to keep him upright before she moved away from him. Thomas positioned himself under the car chassis and prayed for superhuman strength to shift it enough to free him.

'One, two, three…' He braced himself against the heavy weight, pushing with everything he had while Daisy ducked under the water. It was difficult to see what she was doing but guessed the moment she pulled the leg free when he heard Jimmy cry out. He knew Daisy would do her best not to jolt his injury any more than she had to and cause him unnecessary pain, but the circumstances were making that a difficult task.

Thomas was doubled over, his hands on his knees, legs shaking with the effort it was taking to keep the weight off Jimmy and Daisy.

Eventually she came back up. Knowing her lack of swimming ability made her endeavour all the more remarkable.

'Pull him as far away from here as possible. I can't hold this up much longer.' His body was spent, fuelled on pure adrenaline to keep them safe.

As soon as they were a suitable distance away he let the car down and dodged out of the way himself.

'Are you okay, Thomas?' Daisy called to him as she helped Jimmy to the back of the house.

Thomas waved, too physically exhausted to speak. Although he couldn't rest when they had a broken leg to tend to.

'We…we have to get him somewhere dry.'

'Where?'

They both looked around the swamped garden and saw the impossible task, with the scrap metal causing obstructions everywhere. He tried the back door and was relieved to find it unlocked, though the kitchen floor was flooded too. The surface of the wooden dining table was dry even if the legs were surrounded by water. He cleared the dirty dishes onto the nearest worktop before going back to fetch the others.

'Do you think you can help me lift him in there?' Thankfully, Jimmy was of slight build, but it was still a big ask, taking into account his injury and how long Daisy had been submerged in the water too.

'I'll do my best, but we should stabilise that leg. Can you reach the medical supplies?' She pointed to the bag she had set on the roof of one of the cars. Thomas retrieved it but he was sure there was nothing in there capable of holding the leg in place to prevent further injury. However, he did have painkillers. After popping a couple out for Jimmy he spotted an old wooden packing crate, bobbing about over by the shed, and grabbed it. With some brute force using his hands and feet, he was able to pull it apart. They hauled Jimmy up the back steps and tied two wooden slats around his leg with bandages to hold it steady. Once they had done their best to limit movement of the injured limb, Thomas grabbed him under the shoulders.

'Okay, Daisy, if you can take the legs we can try and get him inside and up onto the table. Brace yourself, Jimmy.' He tried to take the bulk of the weight and staggered back inside. Jimmy winced but he was a trooper, as was Daisy, managing to lift their patient's lower half.

It was a struggle to get him up onto the table and involved a lot of manoeuvring, pushing, panting and swearing from all three of them.

'Do you have any dry clothes or towels, Jimmy? Those wet things are going to have to come off so we can keep you warm.' Daisy voiced their other concern over him getting pneumonia or going into shock.

'There's stuff upstairs in the airing cup-board.'

While Daisy went in search, Thomas hunted in the drawers for scissors. 'I'll have to cut these clothes off you, Jim. It's important we do this quickly and don't jolt you about too much.'

'Okay.' The weariness was beginning to tell but they had to keep him conscious until they could get him to hospital.

Thomas removed the torn, bloodied trousers quickly. Once Daisy came back, they were able to prop Jimmy's head up on a folded towel and cover him in a warm thick blanket.

'I'll go and see if there's an ambulance on the way.' Thomas left the room to chase up the ambulance on the phone and to see if there were any emergency services in the vicinity.

Firemen were going door to door to evacuate anyone still trapped in their houses and transporting the very young and elderly by dinghy to safety. The paramedics were taking any of those seriously injured or in shock away by ambulance. Thomas managed to flag someone down to explain their predicament. With a lot of expert help, Jimmy was finally stretchered out.

'How are things looking back there?' Thomas asked one of the paramedics, keen for news about any other residents they might have missed.

'There don't seem to be any other serious injuries but obviously the flooding has left a lot of people with nowhere to sleep tonight. The pub has offered rooms, but they're overrun at the minute.'

'What about your place, Thomas? You could put a lot of the residents up until tomorrow, when we find out for sure how bad the damage is. The house should be high enough up on the hill to be unaffected and there's sufficient room.' Daisy was biting her lip as if she knew what she was asking was out of order when he had made it clear how he felt about sharing his space.

His initial reaction was to say no and shoot down the idea before the guilt began to weigh on his mind. It wasn't fair of Daisy to burden him with the responsibility of leaving these people spending the night wet and cold in homes that probably were not fit for habitation in their current state. Yet she had put her fears aside tonight to help Jimmy because her strength was needed in that moment to save the man. Now he had to dig deep in order to help those in need of support. It wasn't going to be easy, but he was sure Daisy would be there for him when they'd been working as a team all night.

'You're right. Tell anyone in need of somewhere to stay to go to Dr Ryan's house. It's the grey one up on the hill.' Thomas gave his permission to the emergency services to direct people to his place, but his stomach was already rolling at the thought of so many traipsing into the family home.

Even though it had been her suggestion, the look of concern on Daisy's face told him she understood what a big deal this was for him. 'Are you sure?'

He nodded. 'These are my friends and neighbours and I'll do whatever I can to help them.'

'After tonight, I doubt anyone would think otherwise.' Her smile was as warm and welcome as a hug, although not as enjoyable as the one they had shared earlier. When he'd been content to hold her, to breathe her in as long as she would let him.

That comfort, that strength and heart that only came with a connection from another person was something he hadn't had since Jade. A feeling he hadn't realised he was missing until she was gone from his arms again. Thomas didn't know what it was about Daisy that had made him come alive again, but he knew it didn't come around every day.

The problem was that he didn't know what to do about it.

CHAPTER FIVE

DAISY WAS TIRED, her very bones ached, she was soaked through and more than a little bit emotional but, with Thomas still ploughing on, she knew she had to do the same. He had insisted on stopping off at her place before driving back to his house. Thankfully his car had survived the storm, even if it was a little battered.

'Are you positive you're okay to do this?' He was checking on her emotional state again, as he had been doing continually since they'd left the village, regardless that he was the one about to be tested so far out of his comfort zone with the influx of strangers in his house.

She wasn't used to anyone caring about her enough to ask and the question alone made her well up. To have someone with her during a difficult time meant all the difference after years of coping on her own and trying to stay strong. Thomas's support let her express how she was actually feeling and was healthier than holding everything back for fear of appearing weak. He wouldn't try to take advantage of that vulnerability when he was leaving himself so exposed too and it made her less afraid to let her guard down a little.

Tonight, all he had shown was compassion and generosity, thinking of everyone but himself, when she knew the personal demons he was fighting at the same time.

'There are others who have lost a lot more than I have.'

'That doesn't diminish your loss or make your upset any less important. I can manage alone if you want to take some time out.'

Daisy appreciated his concern but wouldn't have been comfortable sitting doing nothing while he ran around the village in his superhero cape and tights. Besides, she needed to keep busy to take her mind off whatever mess was awaiting her at the cottage.

'I told you, I'm fine.' She gave him a smile she hoped was convincing enough to stop him worrying.

As anticipated, the floodwater had covered the entire ground floor of the cottage, ruining everything in its path. It was a lot to take in, seeing the devastation when she hadn't long moved in.

The rug she'd bought to provide some warmth underfoot when walking on the wooden floors was floating in a sea of dirty water, the once vibrant colours now a muddy brown. Even the dachshund-shaped draught excluder she'd bought from a local craft store, and nicknamed Dex, had doggy-paddled away from his prime spot along the bottom of the door. Now he was buried, only his back end visible, apparently having suffered from some sort of mummification from the pile of sodden magazines which had been swept off her coffee table.

It seemed absurd to have a lump in her throat over such trivial things, but she'd been trying to make this a home. These small purchases and additions to the cottage represented her setting down some roots and tonight that had been taken away from her. Her efforts to fit in, to make a life for herself had been wiped out in a flash. She felt as though she was back in that limbo, with nowhere to really call home.

Not that she would let anyone see her cry over something as pathetic as some ruined soft furnishings. She was stronger than that now. At least on the outside.

'No offence, but I didn't like the choice of décor anyway. It will give me a chance to re-decorate to my own taste.'

'I can see you've tried to put your own stamp on the place already. I'm so sorry about everything you've lost.' Thomas put an arm around her shoulders in sympathy and it was all she could do not to bury her head in his chest and sob when he was offering her some much-needed emotional support.

'The insurance should replace anything you need to get the place back to how you want it, Daisy. Obviously we'll have to wait until we get the place dried out first.'

For Daisy, it wasn't about the monetary value of the items destroyed; it was the time and joy that had gone into choosing those things, in trying to make a home for herself. Little Morton was the first place she'd put any effort into that kind of thing. As though this was the one place where she could see herself settling down. Belonging. This was a reminder that nothing for her was certain, and she didn't have family to help her pick up the pieces.

'There's not much we can do about it in the meantime so we should probably go and see to your house guests,' she said, keen to get away from the sight of her life here in ruins. Thomas's house was about to become her welcome refuge for the night too.

Thomas had ferried as many people as he could to his house in his car and had instructed the emergency services to send anyone else there who needed a place to stay. The fire brigade was working hard to move any large obstructions in the area and pumping water away as best they could. The paramedics were on hand giving hygiene advice to those who might not have been seriously injured but had come into contact with the dirty water. Everything would have been contaminated by the bacteria present in the floodwater and needed to be cleaned thoroughly. The electricity supplier had sent out engineers to make sure the power lines were safe and running after the storm. Everyone was rallying around to repair the significant damage done to the village.

Goodness knew how long it would take to get back to normal. Especially if they had any more rainfall like they had experienced earlier. The clear-up was going to be tough, but at least for now those most affected would have somewhere safe and warm to stay.

As a result, Daisy and Thomas had become the hosts, welcoming people in and providing hot food and beverages. They were in the kitchen now, making tea and coffee with bottled water for the people currently huddled in the living room.

'Where is everyone going to sleep tonight?' Though the house was four times the size of hers, there were more people than bedrooms. She hadn't thought things through properly before volunteering his home as a hotel for the night. Likely because she'd never expected him to agree so willingly. They had only known each other for a short time but Thomas was an inspiration to anyone struggling with their demons when he faced his so heroically. Daisy wished she had the same strength. Then she might not be facing spending the rest of her days alone, afraid of history repeating itself and burning her in the process.

'I'll put the young families in the bedrooms and hopefully the rest will bed down where they are. There should be enough blankets and pillows for everyone to have a makeshift bed at least.' If he was indeed fazed by having his home invaded by so many at once, he wasn't showing any visible sign of discomfort. Probably for her benefit and those who'd been invited to stay. Daisy was impressed that he was capable of setting aside his personal issues for the sake of others, when not so long ago he'd been stressing over one stranger arriving in his village.

He had mellowed from the man who had 'greeted' her on her arrival to the village. That barrier protecting him from people like those who had hurt his father was gradually lowering and Thomas was doing his best to make everyone feel at ease instead of pushing them away.

Daisy distributed the drinks and whatever snacks she could find in the kitchen to the house guests dispersed throughout the reception rooms on the ground floor of the family home. It was a huge, imposing building filled with the history of previous generations. The wooden panelling on the walls made the house seem even more dark and imposing. Thick rich red carpeting underfoot gave the place a regal air, along with the gold-plated fixtures and fittings. It was no wonder Thomas was paranoid about letting people in when the place felt like a museum. So many precious heirlooms were dotted about which probably should have been behind glass for protection. It would only take one errant child or a clumsy visitor to shatter the Chinese vases or porcelain figures and a piece of history could be lost for ever.

Despite the portraits of his ancestors frowning at any intruders from the walls, Daisy could see how lonely Thomas could be here, miles away from village life. There were no neighbours, no noise outside and he likely only inhabited a fraction of the large dwelling. It reminded her of her London apartment, only on a much larger scale.

Hopefully he could take something positive away from tonight's events too, seeing the house come alive with people, laughter and chat. With any luck it wouldn't be for the last time. He was clearly a much loved, well-respected member of the community and Daisy knew if Thomas would let people in they would gladly include him in the whole of village life. She could only dream of the same. Perhaps then they wouldn't seem to be each other's only lifeline.

There were lots of pats on the back and words of gratitude uttered to Daisy and Thomas as they did their best to make everyone comfortable. He came to her empty-handed after handing out bedding to their exhausted neighbours.

'Is there anything left for me or should I curl up in the bath for the night?' She was only half joking. As much as she was longing for a bed, she would sleep anywhere right now.

'I thought you could sleep in my room.'

Her eyebrows shot up at the presumption. 'Excuse me?'

Thomas at least looked embarrassed when she queried his proposition. 'I mean, you can take the bed. I'll take the floor. I know I should give up my room for someone else but I'm not ready to leave strangers alone with my personal items.'

There was a warm glow inside her at the thought that he was happy for her to have entry into his inner sanctum. He no longer saw her as an unwanted stranger.

'In that case, take me to your bed, Your Grace.' She couldn't help but tease him when he looked so adorably ruffled. Up until now she hadn't seen him as anything other than confident and cool in his actions. Perhaps she wasn't a totally safe option after all if she could manage to get him a tad flustered before bedtime.

They walked up the stairs in silence to his bedroom, as though they were expecting something major to happen. Daisy knew that wasn't a possibility, not just because there was so much else going on here tonight, but also because neither of them was ready for any romantic entanglement. They were two broken souls who had simply found some comfort together. Now they had to be careful they didn't mistake that for anything more dangerous.

Thomas opened his bedroom door and let her walk in first. It was such a stark contrast to the rest of the house, Daisy could see why he was reluctant to share it with strangers. Gone were the stern faces of previous Earls, replaced with sunny images of the harbour. The furniture was modern but looked comfortable, unlike the expensive pieces she had seen downstairs but had been too afraid to sit on in case she broke something priceless. Thick luxurious carpet cushioned her feet with every step she took into Thomas's domain. It felt homely.

'This is such a lovely room. Why don't you redecorate the rest of the house like this?' She plonked herself on the edge of the super-king-size bed in the middle of the room.

Thomas smiled and closed the door behind him, locking them into their own world away from everyone else for a while. 'I guess I haven't got used to being the owner yet. It feels almost as though I'm merely the caretaker here, looking after someone else's stuff. I wouldn't even know what to do with everything or where to put it.'

'The opposite of my problem.' Her mind

drifted back to the devastation at the cottage and whether or not she would be able to salvage anything.

'We can deal with that tomorrow. It's been a long tiring day and we should both get some sleep. There's bottled water in the bathroom if you'd like to get washed?' Until they could be sure the water was safe to use again, the water company had provided bottles of water for washing and drinking to everyone in the village.

Thomas rummaged in a nearby chest of drawers and pulled out some grey tracksuit bottoms and a T-shirt. 'I know they're not your size or style, but they are dry.'

'Thanks,' she said as he tossed them over to her and she hurried into the bathroom before she embarrassed herself by crying or, worse, by making an unwanted advance.

It would be easy to give in to that urge to hug him, to kiss him when he had been her strength tonight. He had been everyone's strength, yet she knew he wouldn't expect anything from anyone in return. It wasn't something she was used to. In her experience when people, men in particular, provided her with security she was expected to hand over her independence in gratitude. Tonight she would have gladly done so, uncaring of the consequences, if it meant she could let go of that tight control of her emotions and let Thomas look after her for a while.

She washed sparingly with the cold water from the bottle provided. They had left enough downstairs for their guests to do the same.

By the time she had dried off and dressed in his too big, comfy clothes, he had bedded down on the floor with the array of cushions which had been decorating the bed.

'I'll just go and brush my teeth then I'll turn the light off.' He disappeared into the bathroom, but not before Daisy had a peek at his half-naked form.

It was just as well she was climbing into bed before she swooned at the flash of toned torso and tight buttocks encased in jersey fabric as he left the room. She lay down and attempted to force herself to sleep. Impossible now she had seen that body, which had been teasing her ever since the festival. Okay, so she was attracted to him. Big deal. Most people in the village likely had a crush on the rich, handsome doctor who had come to the rescue tonight. It didn't mean anyone was going to act on it, including her. Even if it was torture lying in his bed, knowing he was so close.

As promised, he turned the light off once he had finished brushing his teeth and she heard the rustle of cushions as he tried to get comfortable.

'Night,' she said into the darkness.

'Night, Daisy.'

It was impossible to say how long she lay there, wide awake, replaying the events of the evening in her mind. As exhausted as she was, sleep was elusive because of the drama and the personal loss she had suffered. Not to mention the awareness that Thomas was lying in his boxers on the floor beside her. The intermittent sound of him plumping the cushions and tossing and turning finally became too much for her.

'You know this bed is big enough for the two of us to sleep in without being in the same postcode. We're both adults, Thomas. I think we can manage to share without making a huge deal about it.' She didn't want him to think she was making a move on him. It was simply the guilt from having this huge bed to herself which had prompted the suggestion.

'Are you sure? I can't seem to get comfortable here.'

'I noticed,' Daisy grumbled as the mattress dipped and Thomas slid in beside her.

'You can't sleep either?'

'Nope. Too much going on in my head to switch off, unfortunately.' A matter which was not going to be helped now he was lying next to her. If she turned onto her side there was a possibility of coming into contact with his warm, partially naked body and that temptation alone was enough to keep her awake.

'It's been a weird day all right.'

'In the hope I don't sound too condescending, I want to say I'm proud of you for letting everyone stay here tonight. I know that was a huge leap of faith for you.' She saw the glint of his smile through the darkness.

'Thanks. Although I'm not sure there was much choice. I couldn't leave everyone else to fend for themselves.'

'No, but considering everything that's happened in the past, I know it can't have been easy.'

'It wasn't and not simply because I've opened up the house to people.'

Daisy heard a movement and a tilt of her head found him staring into her eyes.

'Oh.' She held her breath, afraid to interrupt his train of thought, and waited for him to open up some more.

'The men who broke into the house and assaulted my father were strangers to us but not to my girlfriend at the time. Jade was a volunteer at a charity I started. I thought I should take a leaf out of my father's book and commit my time and money to a worthy cause. I was doing it for all the right reasons, I thought. I wanted to make a difference to those who, through no fault of their own, didn't have the same opportunities in life I had.'

That was a leaf straight out of his father's book, helping the less fortunate for no other reward than knowing he was doing the right thing, and Daisy had to commend him for that.

'What happened?'

'Jade became a big part of my life. Of course that meant taking her home, introducing her to my father and sharing my life with her. It never occurred to me that I was being played. That it was all a scam, a set-up to find out as much about my family and our finances as possible. She waited until I was away from home before making her move. Unknown to me, she was sharing all those details about my life with her nefarious friends. She stopped by the house, my father invited her in, unaware she had brought a criminal gang with her. I was so wrapped up in myself, in Jade and in getting my project off the ground, I was blind to the danger waiting out there. I brought it home with me.' The pain and guilt in Thomas's voice was difficult to listen to. It was raw, without self-pity, only regret.

'That's terrible. Such a betrayal on so many levels.'

'It's not your fault. If anything, I should be apologising to you for taking out my issues on you when you first arrived.'

'I survived, didn't I? As it happens, I was trying to lay some ghosts of my past to rest too.' She had never shared the details of those troubled years with anyone except Thomas's father but here, under the cover of darkness, having a heart-to-heart with Thomas, it felt safe to share.

Another deep breath. 'Where to start? I never knew my dad. I think he and my mum were passing ships in the night. She married when I was nine but took off a year or so later, leaving me with my stepfather and step-brothers, who treated me like their personal servant.'

'A real-life Cinderella?'

'I never thought of it that way, but in some ways I suppose so.'

'Didn't social services get involved?'

'I was too terrified to tell anyone what was

going on at home. I'd been threatened not to open my mouth or I would end up in a children's home, which sounded scary to a young girl who already felt alone in the world. Besides, my stepfather could have charmed anyone. From the outside he seemed like a respectable family man, because that was what he wanted people to think. No one would have believed the monster he was at home. His sons were no better. They were teenagers who should have been capable of looking after themselves or standing up for me, but they were carbon copies of him and enjoyed making my life hell. Your father was a little like my Fairy Godfather. At the time of applying for his scholarship I was living with my boyfriend, Aaron, which wasn't much better than the house I'd left. He was controlling, didn't like me going out and didn't want me working. I was completely dependent on him and I thought I had to be grateful for it. Then I saw an article about the scholarship your father was offering and I knew it was my way out. Since then I've worked hard to keep that independence he helped me achieve. I owe him so much and I'm truly sorry I'll never get to tell him that in person.' It choked her up that he had been so cruelly taken away from both of them. Of course it was a huge loss to

Thomas not having his father, but Daisy felt it too when he had helped her take back her power.

'He was one of a kind all right. Too soft-hearted for his own good. I was afraid you were taking advantage of him.'

'I got that. You didn't know me and I suppose you were just looking out for your father. I like to think we were friends at the end and that's why he told me about the position at the medical centre. I had recently split up with someone and was keen for a new start. He always seemed to appear when I needed him most.'

'He talked about you a lot and how proud he was of everything you'd achieved. Bringing you here was his way of telling me "I told you so" when I became cynical about these strangers he was helping.' Thomas laughed. It was a warm comforting sound Daisy wanted to snuggle into.

'He'd be proud of everything you've done in the village.' It was plain to see Thomas's devotion to his family's legacy went far beyond his title and property. The people of Little Morton were his family now, but he just couldn't see it.

'He deserved better than he got. You don't know the half of what he went through and still put everyone else's needs first. Even my mother treated him badly. She cheated on him with the gardener—so cliché—then cleaned out their joint bank account. Thankfully, the majority of his money was tied up in investments and was too difficult for her to get at, otherwise she would probably have left him destitute. We never saw her again. Anyone else would have tightened their hold on their wallet, but not my father. He poured all of his love and money into his charitable projects after that.'

'Am I one of his charitable projects?' she asked with her tongue firmly in her cheek.

'You are his greatest success.'

Daisy turned onto her side so they were mere centimetres away from each other. 'I think that honour goes to his high-achieving, caring son.'

Although it sounded cheesy as they formed their mutual appreciation society, Daisy meant every word of it. The Earl might be gone, but he had raised this beautiful man who had come along just when she'd needed him. Her life had not been lonely since she'd set foot in the clinic and crossed paths with Dr Ryan.

All of a sudden the room seemed more intimate, the space between them minute, and the air filled with crackling anticipation. Daisy knew she should turn away from him and temptation, but she didn't want to. Every second since she'd met Thomas had been leading to this moment. Although she hadn't expected to be sharing his bed tonight.

They were smiling at each other, knowing what was coming next but both wary of making that crucial move. Then Thomas moved across until his head was resting on her pillow and pressed his lips against hers.

Daisy shut her eyes to fully let go of her inhibitions, closed her ears to those voices of doubt trying to spoil it and kissed him back. That first soft pressure appeared to be Thomas seeking permission for more and she willingly granted it. They parted for a mere second before reconnecting, this time with more force and increasing passion.

Daisy's heart was pounding somewhere in her throat as he cupped her cheek with his hand whilst his mouth sought hers again and again. He teased his tongue along her bottom lip before dipping inside.

This was definitely not the buttoned-up Earl she had thought she would be working with.

Arousal was flooding her body the same way the river had crashed through the village, causing just as much devastation. She hadn't come here to get involved with anyone, let alone her work colleague. Yet they had a connection she couldn't ignore, or apparently walk away from.

Thomas slid his hand up under her loose top and palmed her breast, taking a possessive hold which left her gasping at the bold move. It turned her on so much she was a writhing mass of hormones restless for more. She wanted him, wanted his hands all over her body, making her forget everything except how he was making her feel in that moment. Alive, sexy and, most of all, wanted.

Impatience saw her reach for him, being as daring as he had been. She took hold of his hardness through his boxers, enjoying the hiss of air through his teeth as she tested his resolve. The feel of him in her hand was a powerful aphrodisiac, knowing she'd been the one to get him in this state.

'Daisy—' His strained plea only spurred her on to want to please him and make him feel the way she did.

'Hmm?'

'Daisy. Stop.' He grabbed her hand and moved it away.

'What—what's wrong?' She scooted back, giving him some space and trying to distance

herself from the humiliation threatening to
engulf her.

'Do we really want to go here?' His tone
had changed from rampant and ready to re-
gretful, suggesting that he didn't.

'I thought—' Well, she hadn't been thinking or she would have realised what a big
mistake they were about to embark on too.

He was right. Events had completely overtaken them tonight, forcing them together.
They were tired, emotional and seeking comfort and that would never be a good reason
to sleep together. They would only come to
regret it once everything went back to normal. Their lives had been turned upside down
and now they were clinging to something familiar and comforting like sex to save them
from drowning.

'Tonight has shaken us both up and we're
not thinking clearly. Are we really ready to
start something, Daisy?'

'When you put it like that...' His words
were enough to throw cold water over the previously sizzling sheets. To Daisy, a relationship of any kind entailed giving up who she
was to please someone else, compromising
her life to accommodate a partner's wishes.
She hadn't come all this way to repeat those
mistakes.

'I didn't think so. Should I move back onto the floor?' Thomas kicked off the covers, ready to scramble away from her.

She didn't want him to think she couldn't control herself around him. 'There's no need. Honestly. Point made, loud and clear.' Doing her best not to take offence or let him think she would attempt to seduce him in the night, Daisy punched one of her pillows into a makeshift barrier between them. There would be no inadvertent touching or straying into temptation now. It was unlikely there would be any sleeping either, now she knew exactly what Thomas could arouse in her. Just one look, one word from him and her mind would bring her straight back into his bed. Where lips were clashing, bodies were writhing and that thrill of anticipation made her feel more alive than she had in years.

It would have been easier to keep working alongside each other if she had let him keep resenting her instead of lusting after him, yearning for the release they had just denied each other.

Whether they had slept together or not, they would never look at each other the same way again. Damn it if Daisy didn't want him to feel the same way she did and to hell with the consequences. In that moment she would

have quit her job if it meant one hot night together. Then there would be no relationship
worth worrying about. Except she would still
be giving up her life for a man. She simply
couldn't win.

CHAPTER SIX

THOMAS ROSE IN the early hours of the morning. He had to before the last of his restraint gave way with Daisy lying next to him in bed. Last night had been a close call and he wondered if he regretted not giving in to the desire to make love to her more than if he had.

Goodness knew he wanted nothing more than to have her completely naked in his arms, but damned common sense had just about managed to override his natural instinct. The moment she had touched him back he'd realised the implications of taking that next step.

Never mind that they still had to work together, but they had just opened up to one another about why they were so unsuited as a couple. Neither were ready to trust again or share their lives with anyone. That would never be a good basis for a relationship and, being in such close proximity, a fling was not a possibility. Nor was it likely they could have one night together and then he would simply walk away and forget about it. It was going to be difficult enough putting their passionate encounter behind them and carrying on as though nothing had happened.

With so many house guests, he thought it prudent to make a start on breakfast or at least set out enough food for people to help themselves. Whatever it took to kill time before they were able to survey last night's damage in the daylight.

He pulled on his shirt and trousers in case he offended any ladies from the village he might run into. It was also his way of calling time on sleeping next to Daisy.

She was fast asleep, looking very much at home in his bed. The room must have become too hot for her in the night; now she was lying on top of the covers, his joggers discarded on the floor. Her T-shirt-cum-nightdress was riding high on her thighs and corrupting his thoughts.

Ignoring his horny inner demon, he left the room and the delectable sight of Daisy sprawled across the pillows to deal with the needs of the others who had stayed the night. Those who were easier taken care of and didn't leave him worrying about the aftermath. At most, the only trouble there would be downstairs was a lack of food and extra housework when everyone had gone.

Neither he nor Daisy had eaten last night, too busy making sure their friends and neighbours had enough to keep them comfortable for the night. As a result he was ravenous and in need of a caffeine fix. He briefly contemplated making some breakfast for Daisy, but walking back into that room and seeing her in his bed again would be asking for more trouble. It would be better to leave her until daylight and let her help herself. To breakfast and nothing else.

Despite trying to be as quiet as possible so he didn't disturb anyone, Thomas thought he heard someone moving about upstairs. He prayed Daisy hadn't wakened and decided to follow him down. It would defeat the whole purpose of him escaping the sexual tension between them.

He waited, listening for the sound of footsteps on the stairs but none came. Then a shrill cry pierced the silence and Thomas was bounding up the stairs in his bare feet, taking as many as he could at once.

His thoughts were only of Daisy, concerned she might have hurt herself in the dark, and he cursed himself for leaving her alone. When he reached the communal landing, the commotion seemed to be coming from the opposite end of the hallway to his bedroom, in one of the spare rooms. Daisy appeared in the doorway of his room, hair flattened on one side, wiping sleep from her eyes.

'Thomas? What's wrong?'

'I don't know. I thought you'd hurt yourself.'

She shook her head. 'Whoever that was woke me up. I was fast asleep. I didn't even hear you get out of bed.'

The pointed look accusing him of taking the coward's way out didn't go unnoticed by Thomas but that was a discussion which could wait. Another anguished cry sent them both rushing towards the source. One of the guest bedroom doors was wide open, a man he recognised as one of his patients frantically pacing the room with his phone clamped to his ear.

Thomas gave a polite knock on the door to make him aware of their presence. 'Is everything all right, Neil? We thought we heard someone in pain.'

The man threw up his hands. 'I was just about to come and find you, Doc. Janine is in labour and no one can tell me when an ambulance can get here.'

A lowing sound came from the en suite bathroom and Daisy rushed in first to give assistance.

'How far apart are the contractions?' Thomas asked as she gained admittance to the bathroom.

'They're coming fast. Too fast.' There were already dark shadows beneath the father-to-be's eyes. Clad only in his underwear and white as a sheet, his wife's labour seemed to have come as big a shock to him as everyone else.

'She's almost full-term, isn't she?' It wouldn't be surprising if the ordeal the couple had been through, with the flood and the potential loss of their home, had started labour prematurely. Something which would have ideally been dealt with in a hospital environment but here, with no real idea of when help would arrive, they wouldn't be equipped to deal with any possible complications.

'Thirty-six weeks. We don't even have her bag here or anything for the baby.' The anxious father dropped down onto the mattress, apparently overwhelmed by the occasion and it was little wonder.

Thomas wondered how much of their baby's belongings had even survived the water damage. Although he was sure the community would rally around to make sure the family had all they needed. The most important thing now was to make sure this baby arrived safely.

As another contraction made itself known to the mother and the rest of the household, Thomas knew that job was going to be down to him and Daisy. Even in these difficult circumstances, he was sure their working partnership would prove more successful than their personal one.

'Thomas? You need to get in here.' Daisy's urgent tone drew him into the bathroom straight away. She was kneeling on the floor beside Janine, who was holding her hand so tightly it looked as though she had cut off the circulation.

'Can't you give her something?' Neil, unable to bear his wife being in distress, was practically begging them to do something for her.

'I'm sorry, it's too late to give her any pain relief,' Daisy added.

'Can she hold on until the paramedics get here?' Thomas kept his voice low so as not to startle the couple.

Daisy shook her head. 'This baby is coming now.'

'Do you have any experience assisting a

birth?' he asked, prepared to let her take the lead if she had more expertise in this area. The last time he had assisted in a birth had been during his first year at the clinic. A patient had gone into labour during a snowstorm and he and his father had been able to reach her before an ambulance could. He'd had his father to guide him then, the man who had been present at most of the births of the locals over the years.

'Not since medical school,' Daisy said, a faint flicker of uncertainty in her eyes before she returned her attention to Janine, who was crying out as another contraction hit. Thomas knew Daisy would step up and do what needed to be done for her patients, just as he would. They worked well together, so he had no doubt they could do this between them.

'In that case, we'd better get organised.' He rolled up his sleeves before grabbing all the fresh towels he could find from the cupboard.

'You can't deliver our baby here. Can't you at least get her over to the bed?' The worried partner was hovering in the doorway, the compact bathroom too small to house them all.

Thomas understood the need to make her comfortable, to make the birth special, but circumstances had overtaken them. 'I'm sorry but we can't move her now. It's too late.'

'The baby's head is crowning.' Daisy moved into a prime position so she could see what was happening, with Janine panting hard and apparently ready to push.

Thomas knelt down on the floor. 'Okay, Janine, big deep breaths and when the next contraction hits I want you to push as hard as you can.'

The frightened woman nodded back at him, trusting that he knew what he was doing. In truth, he hadn't delivered a baby in a very long time, but it looked as though Janine had done most of the hard work already.

Daisy poured some cold water from one of the bottles the water company had distributed onto a flannel and laid it on the woman's forehead to try and cool her down. 'That's it, big deep breaths. You're doing so well, Janine.'

The expectant father was pacing up and down the room but keeping an eye on the proceedings. Janine's breathing suddenly became quicker, panting through another contraction.

'With this one I need you to bear down, and I'll be here to catch Baby, okay?' He gave what he hoped was a reassuring smile even though his heart was pounding hard and he was beginning to perspire.

Everyone needed to have confidence in him to deliver this baby safely, and he had to push away his own fears to believe it himself.

Janine cried out as she squeezed Daisy's hand when the next contraction hit hard.

'Good girl. You can do this.' Although Daisy was talking to their mother-to-be, Thomas took the positive statement for himself. He could do this too.

With the towels covering the cold tiled floor, he got ready for the baby to slither out. Except when the head emerged, panic began to set in that perhaps he was out of his depth after all.

'Janine, I need you to stop pushing for a while and take long deep breaths.'

Daisy immediately turned to see what was wrong. 'The umbilical cord is wrapped around baby's neck so we need you to slow things down until the doctor can release it.'

The matter-of-fact way Daisy delivered the news kept Janine calm during a time which could have been potentially life-threatening for the baby. It was up to Thomas to unwrap the cord from the baby's neck before it cut off the blood flow and oxygen supply, causing long-term brain damage or worse.

He was breathing more heavily too as he deftly worked to undo the thick cord. As soon as he was sure the baby was out of danger, he gave Janine the go-ahead to continue pushing. He caught the baby quickly and wrapped him in a clean towel to keep him warm. With his little finger Thomas made sure the airway was clear and gave him a quick check-over to make sure everything was okay.

'Congratulations. You have a lovely, healthy baby boy.' He laid the infant on his mother's chest, welling up himself as she sobbed happy, exhausted tears.

'A boy?' Neil, looking relieved it was all over, appeared beside them.

'Come on in, Dad, so you can get a cuddle too.' Daisy scooted aside so the parents could coo over the baby together.

When she caught Thomas's eye he could see she was teary too, understandable when things could have turned out so differently. She probably felt as he did—relieved that everything was okay and happy for the couple about to embark on the new chapter of their life together as a family.

Although he had no doubt that if further complications had arisen Daisy would have assisted him in their improvised delivery suite. She was every bit as confident and capable as him, and great at keeping people calm in a crisis, including him.

Despite running out on her in the early hours, he was glad she had been there with him. Getting involved romantically would be a complication they could both do without, but Daisy was becoming quite a fixture in his life these days and he wasn't complaining. It felt good to be in company again, to share the wonderful and difficult events with someone who understood the importance of his work. Where most women he had been with inevitably got tired of coming second to his job, Daisy lived her life the same way he did. If a relationship had been something he would ever think about again, she would have been his perfect woman.

It was a touching scene, Janine's head lying on her husband's shoulder as they marvelled at the new life they had created, and Daisy couldn't help but think of the family she would never have. If she couldn't trust another man she wouldn't bring a child into the world and into an unstable environment.

Thoughts of Thomas automatically flitted into her head when he was the only man she had let close in a long time, but recreating this happy little scene was merely a fantasy. Both she and Thomas had been left too scarred by their pasts to entertain the idea of sharing their lives again.

It was a pity. She loved children and could tell by Thomas's kind heart and generous nature he would make a good dad some day. He'd certainly had the right role model in his own father. Maybe Thomas would go on to have a family with someone, but it wouldn't be her. Not when he wasn't even willing to share a bed with her for one night.

When she'd woken up, she'd expected to find him still in bed beside her. Although he'd rejected any idea of sleeping with her, she'd liked the thought of waking up next to him, so she wasn't alone on a night like this. Even that had apparently been too much for him to contemplate. She was going to have to accept he wasn't interested in anything other than a working relationship. No matter how much of a slap to the ego that was to her.

The coloured lights flashing in through the window and onto the ceiling signalled the arrival of the ambulance. 'Looks like the cavalry has arrived.'

'I'll go and direct them up to the room.' A relieved-looking Thomas went to meet the paramedics. She was grateful to have them here too so they could monitor Janine while delivering the placenta.

Daisy and Thomas hovered nearby as the crew carried out their checks on mother and baby. Once they were stretchered out, wrapped up in blankets to protect them from the cold, the tension finally left Daisy's body. They had handed over responsibility to the local hospital now, who would carry out further precautionary measures to ensure all was well before discharging the family back home.

'Well, it's been an eventful day and night, hasn't it?' Daisy made Thomas chuckle as they waved the ambulance off at the front door.

'That's one way of putting it. I wonder if it's safe to try and go back to sleep for a few hours?'

'I'm too wired to sleep now. Though I should probably go back inside where it's warm.' She was still dressed in his oversized shirt and little else.

'Yes, go and put some clothes on. I can't afford to have a staff member down with the cold when the clinic will be chaos after the flooding.' He shooed her away but not before she turned back with one last thing to say.

'Congratulations, by the way, Dr Ryan. It's reassuring to me and everyone else that you're confident in a crisis. It could've been a bit hairy back there so, in case no one else says it, well done.'

Daisy was shivering as she went back into the house, but she had thought it important for Thomas to know he was appreciated and not on his own. Being a doctor could be a lonely profession at times, but she suspected more so for him now his father wasn't around to share the workload or the experiences.

They had just witnessed one of life's miracles together. Thanks to Thomas. Given the conditions, the birth could have been more traumatic, but he had proved yet again he was someone who could be relied upon. That was more important to her than a meaningless fling or giving in to temptation for one night and jeopardising her career and her new life here in Little Morton.

With that in mind, she went back upstairs to put on the pair of baggy joggers he had given her. From now on she was going to remain professional around him and set aside whatever attraction she felt towards him. It was the only way she could move forward and stop driving herself crazy.

'You're just in time. Tea's ready.' Daisy poured two cups of hot, sweet tea. They needed it after the morning they had already had.

'Thanks.' He took a long sip and sighed.

Thomas was bound to be exhausted when he hadn't slept at all. At least she had managed forty winks before their extra guest's premature arrival.

'I'll call later and see how mother and baby are doing, but they both seemed in good health all things considered.'

'I hope there are no more surprises. I don't think I can take much more.' He pulled a chair out from the kitchen table and sat down with his cup of tea.

'Judging by tonight's performance, I would say you can deal with anything thrown at you.' Daisy took her cup and joined him at the table, trying to keep her voice low so as not to wake anyone else. Although all the commotion had stirred a few of the visitors, the house remained reasonably quiet.

'You were with me through everything, Daisy. I didn't do it on my own.' He wouldn't accept her praise without a fight.

'Yay us.' She clinked her cup to his in celebration, bringing a smile to his lips.

They sat in silence for a few moments drinking their tea before Daisy blurted out what had been bugging her since she had woken up.

'Why did you leave the bedroom? And your bed, with me in it?'

Thomas set his cup down, taking his time to formulate an answer. He could have lied to her and say he had heard Janine long before they had known what was happening.

Instead, he said, 'Because I knew it was the only way I'd be able to keep my hands off you.'

His voice was gravelly, as though he was struggling with the inner turmoil of that decision. She knew because she felt the same. Everything in her body had said to give in to the chemistry but her head kept telling her it would be a bad idea. That didn't stop the wanting.

The thought of what could have happened if he had not listened to his inner voice gave Daisy that fluttery feeling she thought she had long since grown out of.

'Would it be such a terrible thing?' Her own voice was husky, full of desire and what-ifs.

'Probably not. Which is exactly why I need to keep my distance.' He was grinning and she was sure he was just as frustrated as her, even if common sense was winning out for now.

He had made his position clear, and Daisy

wasn't going to resort to begging simply to scratch that itch when she knew he was right. It didn't mean she would let the subject lie altogether.

'Didn't the sight of the new family tonight make you think about marriage and children at all?' A person would have to be made of stone not to have been moved by bringing a new life into the world and she was sure it had at least made him think about what it would be like. Just as she had.

'I let you share my bed for one night and you're already talking about marriage and babies? Wow. You're a fast mover.'

She rolled her eyes at his teasing, knowing he was avoiding the subject. 'I'm being serious, Thomas.'

'It's very special being part of something like that but, personally, it doesn't change anything for me. Bringing home people I've known and lived beside for years was a huge step for me tonight. I can't see how I'll ever get over the betrayal and hurt my father and I both suffered. Call it self-preservation if you like, but I don't think it's worth jeopardising everything I have to risk my heart on someone else. I simply can't see myself getting past that to settle down with someone.' His half-smile said it wasn't a decision he had made lightly or easily and he was aware of what he was sacrificing to protect himself. Daisy understood when she was guilty of the same.

However, she believed in Thomas's case it was the burden of unnecessary guilt which was preventing him from living his life to the fullest.

'Does this mean you're considering putting an ad out there for a significant other, with a view to having babies in the future?' He turned the question back on her when she'd been trying to work out what was going on in his head. Daisy hadn't been prepared to share the contents of hers.

'I'm not really in a position to think about that, but you've got this big house, the medical practice and the whole village. Wouldn't you like to share that with someone? To have an heir to carry on the family's good work?' She wasn't volunteering for the position, but she was certain his father wouldn't have been happy that Thomas was using his death as an excuse to stop him getting close to anyone else.

Although the picture of the perfect family was fresh in her memory, it seemed little more than a fantasy to someone who was currently homeless and intentionally single. She had never considered things like marriage and motherhood a possibility when she had shut herself off from the rest of the world as an act of self-preservation. It wasn't as though she had parents who had shown her either were a good idea. Now she couldn't help but wonder what it would be like to have those things with someone like Thomas, who had a loving father to emulate. Who had shown her what it was to have support and work together as a team. Things she was sure were essential in a marriage. If it was ever a notion she would have been willing to give up her independence for, Thomas would have made the ideal husband and father.

He shrugged. 'Of course I would like it. In an ideal world I'm sure you would want that too. I'm simply saying I can't see it happening now. I'm too busy with work and keeping the village on its feet. The clear-up after the flood is going to take some work. I've more than enough to keep me from being lonely, don't worry. Anyway, I wouldn't inflict the upkeep of this place on you or anyone else. When I'm gone, there will be a board appointed to make all the decisions about the house and the village.'

So he had at least thought about it. More than she had, if she was honest. It had been easier to block out things like marriage and babies rather than face up to the fact that those things might not be compatible with her solitary lifestyle. She didn't want to compromise who she was for anyone after fighting so hard to establish a life where she wasn't indebted to anyone. Her Cinderella role wasn't one she intended to return to, ever. Regardless of Prince Charming living all alone in his castle.

It would take more than a glass slipper and the promise of a happy ever after to convince Daisy that fairy tales could come true.

CHAPTER SEVEN

THOMAS WOKE ALONE in bed some hours later, after Daisy had convinced him to get some sleep while she oversaw breakfast for the masses. He would have protested except for the weariness which had overtaken his body and the prospect of the busy day ahead. The needs of the village and its residents would require all the strength he could muster in the aftermath of the flood.

There was a soft knock on the bedroom door. 'Thomas? Are you awake?' It was Daisy calling him softly.

'Yes. Come on in.' He sat up in bed and raked his hand through his hair in an attempt to make himself more presentable.

Daisy emerged, carrying a tray of tea things and what smelled like a cooked breakfast. His stomach rumbled and he realised it had been an age since he'd eaten anything. Even if he had drunk his weight in tea over the past twenty-four hours.

'I brought you some breakfast. Everyone else has been fed and is heading back into the village to see what can be done.'

'You didn't have to do that. Although I am starving.' He took the tray with gratitude and set to work filling his belly with bacon and eggs.

As he tucked in, he was aware of Daisy's lingering glance at his bare chest, which only increased his hunger for more than breakfast. It wasn't easy putting last night behind him when she kept staring at him as though she was ready to jump into bed beside him again.

'Was there enough food for everyone? Did you manage to get anything to eat yourself?' he asked, attempting to distract them both from the half-empty bed where she had lain only hours earlier.

'I did. Queenie brought some more supplies from the corner shop and helped me cook for everyone.'

'That's very kind of her. I'll pay for it all, of course, and thank you, Daisy, for covering for me. I should get up and do my own inspection of the village.' He took another bite of toast and gulp of tea before throwing the covers back.

Daisy's eyes flitted everywhere, as though she didn't know where to look. He wasn't naked, but he might as well have been by the way she was reacting. It amused him that she was acting so coyly when she had been anything but shy in bed with him before he'd had an attack of conscience and called a halt to their fun. He got out of bed and stretched, enjoying the lustful look it drew from his audience.

Yes, he had been the one to put an end to things last night before they went too far, but that didn't mean his ego didn't enjoy a little boost every now and then.

'I…er… I'll let you get dressed, then I'll go with you to see what's needed in the village.' She scurried back out of the door, pretending she hadn't done more than just look last night. He could still feel where she had touched him, the memory growing stronger by the second.

Even without laying a finger on one another they were still able to drive each other crazy. However, he wasn't helping himself get over his wayward fantasies about Daisy. It seemed, no matter his good intentions or his determination to remain unaffected by her, his thoughts, feelings and very actions were driven by Daisy. He was a lost cause but simply too afraid of getting hurt to admit it.

No one would ever have guessed Thomas had been up at dawn that morning delivering a baby by the way he had taken charge of the clean-up operation. He had contacted the insurers to have the damage assessed, then set to work repairing it.

'I have a professional crew coming to help clear the debris, along with those the council has appointed, and I've hired skips to dump whatever rubbish has been accumulated in the street. Hopefully, with everyone working together, we can get the job done twice as fast.'

Along with the people he had hired, Thomas had done his own share of the heavy lifting of broken tree branches and dislodged street furniture. While the rain had stopped long ago and the streets had been dried out by the sun, the devastation left behind was clear for all to see. Everything was covered in a layer of silt and mud. There were cars stranded down by the harbour and though they luckily hadn't been completely submerged it was doubtful they would ever start again.

Daisy had joined the householders doing their best to clear the dirty water from their houses using brooms to push it out as best they could. They were all wearing protective clothing, as advised by the authorities, to prevent any further contamination or infection.

'We should get down to the medical centre and see what the damage is there too.' She caught Thomas as he passed down the street, directing the volunteers who had arrived from the nearby area to help.

'Yes, I suppose so. Are you free to come down and do an inventory with me?'

'Sure.' She handed her broom over to one of the volunteers and steeled herself for whatever they were about to face behind the clinic door.

'You can't put off going home again for ever either,' Thomas reminded her as they dodged the waves of water being cleared out from the doorways.

'Next stop. I promise.' So far she had managed to keep some emotional detachment from everything going on, but she was worried seeing the cottage again would prove too much. In her exhaustion the sight of her new life in ruins might just break the dam.

Thomas was used to seeing the strong Daisy. She didn't want him to witness the fragile version she kept hidden in case anyone tried to take advantage of her again.

'Okay…here goes.' Thomas rolled up the battered shutters and unlocked the door.

Daisy held her breath, waiting for the heartbreak. Once the water had rushed out over their feet and down the hill, she was able to breathe again.

Of course the carpeting was ruined, the walls damp and dirty, but it seemed to be mostly superficial damage so far. They made their way further inside to find the waiting room chairs blocking their way.

'They'll have to be replaced, but that should be easy enough. Once everything is dried out, we'll check the floor is intact, then get the carpet-fitters and decorators in.' He was being practical and logical and it made dealing with the mess that bit easier.

'At least we managed to save the important stuff but it's going to be a while before we can open up again.' It was disheartening to think she had lost her new job as well as her new home, just when she was beginning to feel like one of the locals.

'I'm sure we could set up a temporary clinic up at my house. If it comes to it, you can stay too until your place is ready to move back into.'

'That's a very generous offer—' It showed how far he had come already from the man who hadn't wanted her setting foot in his village only weeks ago. Not to mention inviting patients into his home, which had been his sole sanctuary until last night.

He held up a hand to stop her offering any more thanks. 'Purely selfish on my part. It means you'll be on site whenever you're needed. I would rather you were there than holed up in some hotel miles away from the clinic. It makes sense.'

It did, practically speaking, but, as they'd discovered, they couldn't always rely on common sense to keep them out of trouble. They'd come close to doing something they would have come to regret and if they were working and living together under the same roof there would be no escape from the sexual tension which had a tendency to flare between them.

Once they had cleaned the surgery as much as was possible, they returned to Daisy's cottage to see what could be done there. As they worked to clear out the water and any furniture that was beyond salvaging, Daisy felt the tears she'd managed to hold back the first time stinging her eyes again.

The lack of sleep, manual labour and trauma from the last couple of days finally caught up with her and Daisy burst into loud, messy tears.

'Oh, Daisy, come here.' Thomas clutched her to his chest and she let herself be comforted. She was allowed to be upset and Thomas had already proved he wasn't someone to take advantage of her weakness. Otherwise the two of them would never have left his bed.

The tears stopped long before the embrace ended. She was drawing so much warmth from him she didn't want to let go. It had been a lifetime since she'd been held like this, with someone lovingly stroking her hair and telling her things would be all right. If ever. She had forgotten how it felt to let go of the stress and share her troubles without fear of reprisals. If this had been her ex, he would have used the moment to tell her she was better off with him, that she couldn't cope on her own, reinforcing the idea that she wouldn't be able to manage without someone else's help, leaving her indebted for ever.

Thankfully, those days were behind her and Thomas was nothing like her controlling, manipulative ex. Just as she was no longer the clingy girl with low self-esteem.

Daisy took a step back and wiped her eyes. 'Okay, hysterics over. We've done all we can here. If you don't mind, I'd like to get back to take a shower at your place.' Until she had an expert out to check the electrics, she wasn't sure how safe it was to use her own.

'You'll need to pack some things too.'

'The water doesn't seem to have reached far up the stairs. There's probably no need for me to inconvenience you long-term, Thomas.'

'Don't be silly, Daisy. You can't live upstairs indefinitely, and you could never be an inconvenience. That house of mine is so big I'll hardly notice you're there.' He was doing his best to make this less traumatic for her and she wished it were true.

However, she knew they could be living at opposite sides of his house and her thoughts would still be of him. They managed to disrupt each other's lives without even trying.

'I doubt that… I'll eat all of your food, use all your hot water…'

'And I'll be grateful to have someone share it again. Now, do you want me to come upstairs with you?'

Daisy raised her eyebrows.

'I mean to check things over.' He narrowed his eyes at her, although there was a smile playing on his lips.

She wondered what he would do if she said yes, she wanted him to come upstairs and check her out…

Although he had made it clear he was able to resist everything she had to offer.

'No need. I'm sure it's all fine. I won't be too long. I'd tell you to sit down and make yourself at home but—' She looked around her sodden living room, bare except for the paintings hung high enough on the walls to have avoided the flooding, and another wave of melancholy crashed over her. It seemed she was more invested in this life she had begun in Little Morton than she had anticipated.

Thomas saw the flicker of despair cross her face as she surveyed what was left of her home. While part of him was glad she had become emotionally attached to the place already, he hated to see her upset. After all she had done to help him and everyone else in the village, she deserved a little kindness and happiness herself.

It was said that money couldn't buy happiness, but it could cheer people's spirits when it was used in the right way. He pulled out his phone, aware that cash could also bypass waiting times for deliveries. In fact, on this occasion, he was going to take advantage of his wealth and status for once to get what he wanted. It was for a good cause, and if it

made Daisy smile again it would be worth
every penny and favour he called in.

Daisy was relieved to have left the cottage,
and the dank smell permeating the air within,
to go back to Thomas's house, which seemed
more welcoming in the daylight. It was set
back off a winding driveway, surrounded by
flat green lawns and a protective barrier of
leafy spruces. Plenty of space and privacy for
a young Thomas to play outdoors and have all
the adventures and fun she'd never got to experience, trapped in a childhood of servitude
and fear. Despite their different upbringings,
she was happy he'd had all of this space to explore as a child and hoped his early years had
been relatively normal and happy. She wanted
him to have had some joy in life, when the
last few years appeared to have ground him
down.

'I have a few things to sort out. You know
where the bathroom is, and the water is back
on so just help yourself to anything you need.'

'Thanks.' Daisy was almost relieved to
have some space to herself for a while. Dealing with the carnage at the cottage had been
emotionally exhausting and she was still pro-
cessing her reaction to it and the way she had
let Thomas comfort her. It had been nice to be

held and supported when it felt as if her whole life had just floated away downstream. His presence reminded her there was still something left for her here.

She was glad to have some physical distance from the devastation too, so she didn't have to constantly think about it. At least Thomas's house was warm and dry and free from the havoc which was in evidence everywhere in the village. It was a little oasis of calm and she could see the benefits of hiding away up here, avoiding real life down below. Even if it couldn't be healthy to sustain that detachment on a long-term basis.

She let Thomas go off and do whatever good deeds he had planned to avail herself of his amenities upstairs. It should have felt intrusive letting herself back into his bedroom, using his private bathroom instead of the many she was sure were dotted around the building, but it wasn't. He had invited her into his bedroom and she had found herself enjoying sharing his personal space, getting to know the man behind the family loyalties.

She took her time washing off the trauma of the flood under the hot water before wrapping herself from head to toe in fluffy towels. Her skin was flushed from the heat of the shower, along with her fantasies about

Thomas inadvertently offering himself to her earlier. Left alone with her thoughts and frustrations which lingered from the night before, she had imagined what it would have been like to have him share the shower with her. It was difficult not to think of him in anything other than a romantic light when he had been a hero to the whole village and to her personally.

Not only was he assisting her in the clearup at her home, he had offered her a place in his house for as long as she needed it. A privilege when she knew how greatly he valued his privacy. It was also further proof that he no longer saw her as an outsider. He trusted her not to betray him and she felt embarrassment that she had been sexually objectifying him in response.

It took her some time to unpack her essentials and to pick out a suitable outfit. Although she wanted something practical for whatever physical work was required, Daisy still wanted to look good. After the day she had had it was important to her self-esteem, though she did forgo blow-drying her hair and applying her make-up, which she deemed too frivolous for the current collective mood in the village. She opted for a stylish all-in-one, olive-green boiler-suit, belted at the waist, which still hinted at her curves despite its function as a cover-all.

When she moved to brush her hair at the dressing table, a card propped up against the mirror caught her eye and she smiled, seeing Thomas's familiar doctor scrawl on the gold-edged invitation.

The Earl of Morton requests the pleasure of your company in the garden summerhouse.

 TR

'What are you up to now?' she wondered aloud as she headed downstairs, her curiosity piqued.

Unfortunately, he hadn't left her a map to find her way to the 'summerhouse', which could be anything from an old garden shed to a full botanical garden conservatory.

Everything in this house was a constant surprise to her. From the outside it looked more like a boarding school than a family home. The nondescript grey exterior, complete with standard sash windows, gave nothing away. Stark, stern and functional was how the house presented. Yet inside was a frenzy of colours and clashing patterns. The rooms were smaller than she'd imagined but crammed full of contrasting furnishings and décor. The busy visual of intricately painted ceilings and adorned walls was enough to give her a headache and it seemed as though the layers of Thomas's ancestors had more of a claim on his home than he did.

She navigated her way along the hallway, past the marble busts on plinths and unnecessary velvet drapes on the walls and down the grand staircase. If Thomas was to make his mark on the place, the way she was trying to do in the cottage, she imagined the house would be much more streamlined and bright. He didn't strike her as the sort who liked to show off; he was humble and, despite her previous fears, never lorded his status over anyone.

She kept walking towards the back of the house, through the kitchen where she and Thomas had kept Little Morton's inhabitants fed and watered during the great flood, and let herself out of the French windows onto the patio. Although the paved area and white wrought iron furniture were pristine clean, Daisy couldn't picture Thomas taking the time to sit out here to simply relax or entertain. The magnificent green lawn was interspersed with pink and purple bursts of rhododendrons and camellias and a three-tiered fountain made a beautiful centrepiece. Everything was immaculate and obviously cared for, yet Daisy felt as though she had stepped into a secret garden no one else knew about. It was a shame Thomas kept it all to himself.

She thought about the glamorous garden parties which must have been held here in the past when his ancestors entertained, imagined the sights and sounds of the lawn filled with people and wondered if they would ever happen again. It would be easy to picture herself sitting in the gorgeously ornate swing seat among the blossoms, relaxing and sipping a cocktail. All the things Thomas should be doing instead of treating this place as a museum. She hoped whatever he was up to today was the beginning of him opening up his home as well as his heart to other people.

Since Thomas hadn't given any directions, she followed the stony path winding away from the house, down into the bushy conifer trees at the bottom of the garden. The deeper into the trees she went, the more she felt as though she was walking into a dream.

The sunlight was streaming through the branches, lighting every step leading into a clearing where a small domed building made up of tiny panes of glass sat waiting for her to discover.

'Thomas?' she called out into the ether.

When she got closer she couldn't believe her eyes. The doors to the summerhouse were open and Thomas was sitting at a table beckoning her over. She realised the colourful haze wasn't coming from her rose-tinted glasses but fairy lights hung around the doorframe.

'I thought you needed a treat, as well as something to eat.' He pulled out a chair for her and she drifted to it in a daze.

'How long did I take to get ready?' She couldn't believe he had managed to do all of this in the time it had taken her to shower and get dressed.

'I called in a few favours and waved my credit card around. I had a lot of help putting this together.'

'It's very thoughtful, Thomas, but doesn't it seem in bad taste when the rest of the village is trying to salvage their belongings?' It was such a lovely thing to have done for her, but she was thinking of everyone else out there mopping up.

'All taken care of. I've hired just about every industrial heater there is in the country and brought catering trucks in to feed the residents. If anything, we're the ones missing out.' As he poured her a cup of tea from a china teapot, she knew beyond doubt she was the luckiest person in the village.

'It all looks so inviting.' The porcelain cake stand set in the middle of the table was filled with dainty sandwiches, delicious scones and mini desserts and she couldn't wait to get stuck in.

'I thought we could still have a civilised meal in the midst of all the chaos. Afternoon tea is just what I'm prescribing.' Thomas took a hearty bite from his cucumber sandwich, almost devouring it in one mouthful. This was a man with a healthy appetite and, given her recent graphic fantasies, Daisy wondered if that extended to the bedroom.

She was sure it did. He was a man who thought of everyone before himself. Who liked to give and was generous to a fault.

That tingling sensation started within her again. The one he had encouraged for a short while last night. It was too bad the next time she slept in his house she was liable to be put in the room furthest from his.

Daisy slathered half of her scone with jam and cream before popping some into her mouth, swapping sugar for sex. As yummy as it was, it was no substitute for the handsome man opposite. His kisses were every bit as delicious and moreish as the home-baked goodies on display.

Daisy wasn't sure she was being as civilised as she ought to be for the occasion.

'So, Thomas Ryan rides to the rescue again. The villagers will soon be naming the streets in your honour.' She teased him because it was safer than waxing lyrical about how amazing he was. Everything he did reminded her of that, and she didn't need to be any more enamoured of him. Things were complicated enough between them.

'I'm simply doing what my father would have done. Besides, most of the streets are named after the family anyway. Maybe we could introduce a national holiday in my honour instead.' Every bit as mischievous as she was being, Thomas toasted her with a mini strawberry tart from the top tier.

'I'll be sure to mention it to the relevant people. I think a Thomas Ryan day where we hide away from the rest of the world and eat cream teas might prove popular, you know.'

He stuck his tongue out and threw a strawberry at her. Daisy caught it between her teeth and ate it noisily to rile him.

'We used to do this at home. I remember my mum pouring tea into her best china and cutting into petits fours with a tiny dessert fork.' The wistful look on his face told Daisy it was a special memory and one he was sharing with her today, attaching the same significance to this occasion with her.

'You must miss her. I haven't seen my mum since I was a kid. It was hard carrying on without her. Especially when I never knew my dad. I used to have this dream she'd appear at the school gates some day, scoop me up and take me home with her. I think it was more about getting away from my stepfamily than believing she might miss me or want me back. I don't really remember much about her, to be honest.' The thought of her stepfather or stepbrothers showing up in her life again brought an altogether different reaction to the fore. Anger. Fear. She didn't know whether she would want to slap them for the way they had treated that little girl, lost and alone in the world, or be afraid she would regress to that scared, helpless soul. Either way, she would prefer not to see any of them again.

'Don't get me wrong, I'm not sure I'm in any rush to see my mother again either. I try not to think about her at all because it's so painful to consider how she betrayed my father and walked away from her own son. As you know, it's not something you get over easily. It's just a nice memory I have of all of us together at the dining table as a family.'

Although Thomas had obviously suffered as much as she had emotionally, he painted a vastly different picture from the upbringing Daisy had, where family meals were taken on a tray in front of the television. She'd been the exception, often made to eat in a different room away from the family and, though she'd cooked it, didn't always get the same meals. More often than not, she'd been left to eat the scraps. It was no wonder she couldn't resist a spread like this. She still ate as though she couldn't be sure where her next meal was coming from.

'Hopefully this will be another nice memory to add to that.'

'Every day with you is a treasured moment,' he replied, and Daisy's heart soared a little more.

It should have been one of the worst times of her life and yet Thomas had made it something special. For someone who didn't think it was a good idea for them to get too close to one another, he was going out of his way to spend time with her.

She wasn't the only person in Little Morton he had supplied lunch for or given help to, but she was the only one receiving his individual attention. Despite his protestations, she knew he liked her and as more than a colleague or neighbour she was certain.

She liked Thomas too. For his kindness, his thoughtful ways and for how he had opened up to her. Not every man would be willing to show that vulnerability or be that honest. Indeed, she knew he valued his privacy above most things and sharing that personal information about his mother was a precious gift to Daisy. One she didn't want to let go unnoticed.

'Thank you again, Thomas, for doing this. It was amazingly thoughtful.' She reached across the table and covered his hand with hers.

Thomas looked down at their hands, then back up to her face, his eyes darkening to glittering sapphires as he looked at her. It was clear he had felt that same jolt of electricity she had from that simple touch. They had been through so much together, shared more experiences over the past days than some people shared in a lifetime, and it was unsurprising that they had become closer. Still, the sheer impact of feeling his skin against hers said there was more between them than a working relationship. Something which both scared and exhilarated her at the same time and refused to go away.

Daisy could tell Thomas felt it too by the way he pulled his hand away as though he had been burned. 'It was nothing. I simply wanted to make you smile again.'

He stood up and began to clear away the dirty dishes. Daisy knew he was fighting temptation as much as she was, but it seemed a pointless exercise when they clearly had feelings for one another that went beyond those of mere work colleagues.

She watched him walk back towards the house, drinking in the fine sight of him. The long legs, straight back and cute backside did nearly as much for her as his handsome face and chiselled torso. She'd had a good view when they'd been in bed together and could remember every sexy inch of him.

Her skin was suddenly prickling with a heat only Thomas could bring out on her. She no longer seemed to have control over her own body or emotions when she was around him. An exhilarating but terrifying discovery.

It was a long time since she had taken a risk on anyone and it called for courage and conviction. Perhaps it might be enough to convince Thomas to do the same.

She collected the rest of the dishes and

followed him back up the path and into the kitchen.

'Hey, this is your day off,' he said, with his hands already submerged in soapy water doing the washing-up.

'I don't think I thanked you properly for today.' Daisy wondered if it was the husky tone of her voice which made him abandon his chore to give her his attention.

As he stood there, bubbles clinging to his fingers, she had never been more attracted to anyone in her life. She took one small step towards him, knowing it was a giant leap forward in their relationship. If he rejected her she was in danger of losing everything she had here, but she also knew the time had come to stop denying this attraction and let things play out. Otherwise she could be missing out on the best thing which had ever happened to her simply because of those who had hurt her in the past. Neither her stepfamily or her exes could ever hope to hold a candle to the kind of man Thomas Ryan was. He was a risk worth taking.

Without a word, she reached up, took his face in her hands and kissed him full on the mouth. For a horrifying moment she thought she had got it completely wrong when he didn't respond, his arms still hanging limply by his sides as she clung to him.

Then Thomas was kissing her back, clutching her to him, his wet hands soaking through her clothes, and she didn't care. All that mattered was that they were finally putting their past heartbreak behind them to live in the moment.

A moment which was getting hotter by the second, burning so fiercely Daisy knew there was no way to stop it now. She could only hope when the fire died down she was not left to sift through the ashes for the remnants of the woman she had once been.

Misplaced or not, her faith and her trust were wrapped up in the kiss. Her gift to Thomas for trusting her with the deeply personal insight into his life.

This was a new experience for both of them.

CHAPTER EIGHT

THOMAS HADN'T EXPECTED any of this to happen. His seduction technique didn't usually involve dainty sandwiches and mini éclairs. Something had changed between them and he'd found himself opening up about the pain of his mother leaving, a subject he had avoided even thinking about for decades.

Being with Daisy brought out those memories and emotions because he wanted to be open about who he was with her. Talking to her about the painful things he had experienced in his life helped him work through it, so he no longer attached the same significance to those events. He knew it was because being with Daisy, being his true self with her, was more important than anything else. Although today wasn't supposed to have been about him; he had merely wanted to do something to raise Daisy's spirits. Now he had something else raised in return.

The gentleman in him didn't want to take advantage of her during such a distressing time. Yet the way she was kissing him, her tongue dipping into his mouth to tease and tantalise, wasn't the action of a woman who didn't know her own mind.

A point proved further as she unbuttoned his shirt, pushing it off his shoulders so his body was exposed to her hands and mouth. Thomas inhaled a ragged breath as she kissed her way across his collarbone, circled his nipple with her tongue and tugged on the hardened peak with her teeth.

They had shared a lot over these past days. Danger, trauma, a birth and a bed. It was only natural they should become closer. Especially when the chemistry between them was stronger than ever.

By all accounts, Daisy's past had been as tough as his. Perhaps that was why he longed to make things better for her now. He wanted to see her smile, to help her forget the bad stuff too. Although, right now, when she was doing indescribable things to his body, he simply wanted her.

He wasn't going to ask her again if she was sure this was what she wanted when she was being clear about that. Thomas was the one who had resisted, who had tried to convince them both they could ignore this escalating passion. That exploring it would be worse than letting it pass. He was wrong.

There was nothing in this world which could beat the taste of Daisy on his lips or the feel of her against his skin.

Once Thomas's resolve wavered, all bets were off and so were Daisy's clothes. He had some catching-up to do when she had already tossed his shirt aside and was currently working on his trousers.

'You're beautiful,' he said, genuinely marvelling at the soft white skin of her breasts as he uncovered them, the rosy tips of her nipples he was kneading in his hands. The sight of her alone was enough to make him hard as hell, but having his hands on her made him fit to burst.

'Shut up and kiss me,' she demanded, breathless with impatience.

Thomas didn't have to be asked twice, and Daisy's boldness served to increase his own. His mouth was hard on hers, taking everything she was willing to give. Her arms were wrapped around his neck, pressing her body to his. All soft curves and heat he no longer wanted to resist.

Urgently divesting her of the rest of her clothes, he backed her over to the dining room table. She gasped as he pushed her back onto the hard wooden surface.

'It's cold,' she giggled, sitting up again so her legs were dangling off the edge of the table.

'Sorry.'

'Don't be.' Daisy wound her arms back around his neck and she kissed him so fully, so completely, reminding him it didn't matter where they were. Only that they were together, finally letting themselves revel in this animal passion.

This blinding need to have her was overwhelming, his senses completely overtaken by thoughts of Daisy. He laid her back, kissing her neck, the cleft of her breast, before licking circles around her nipples. When he sucked the pert tips she arched her body off the table.

'Thomas—' The plea to end her frustration as well as his own made him throb until he could hold out no longer.

Although it had been some time since he'd needed one, he kept a condom in his wallet and was glad of it at this moment. In no time at all he had himself sheathed, his wallet and the condom wrapper abandoned on the floor in his haste to get back to Daisy.

Taking his erection in hand, he positioned

himself between her soft thighs and thrust inside her. He let out a groan of satisfaction to match hers and knew immediately that their relationship would never be the same again. This was more than sex when he knew he would give up everything he had just to be with her.

Daisy was a trembling mass of emotions. The foremost of which was absolute ecstasy. Thomas must have kissed every inch of her skin as she was burning everywhere he had touched her. Now their attention was focused entirely on one area, Thomas was as thorough as ever in his ministrations. His hands were digging possessively into her hips as he claimed her again and again. Daisy widened her legs to accept him, hooking them around his waist as he thrust into her once more.

She would never have believed he was capable of such wild abandon, but he was thrusting into her relentlessly, giving them both what they needed at this moment. Sending her hurtling towards that final, thought-obliterating destination. That pressure within her was building so quickly it was beyond her control. All she could do was cling on and enjoy the ride. Literally.

She had a fistful of Thomas's hair in her

hands as her orgasm slammed into her. Her throaty cry echoed through the house, soon followed by Thomas's equally vocal climax.

He collapsed on top of her, panting as hard as she was, trying to catch his breath.

'I hope no one heard us or saw us,' she said, peering over his shoulder at the open back door. An indication of how reckless they had been and how desperate to have one another at any cost.

'There is no one around to bother us and I don't care anyway,' he said, keeping her pinned down with his arms braced either side of her. Not that she was trying to escape when he was kissing her again, his tongue gently probing her mouth and making her wish they were somewhere more comfortable to cuddle together for a while. Now she was coming back down from the clouds, she remembered they were naked in his kitchen.

'You will when your patients start gossiping about that scandalous Dr Ryan who seduced his co-worker on the dining table.'

'I think you might have that the wrong way around.'

Thomas began to dress, hiding that delicious body of his.

'I suppose it does take two to do what we just did,' she conceded, trailing a fingertip seductively down his chest before he covered it completely. Although she had been thinking about this moment for a long time, if she had thought about it properly she would have picked somewhere warmer, where they would still be lying in one another's arms.

All that had been on her mind was that she wanted him to acknowledge the crazy sexy vibes between them. Job done. Now what?

Thomas rested his hands on her shoulders. 'We've been skating around this for days. It was inevitable.'

'And now?' She looked up at him and swallowed hard, waiting in agony for him to tell her if he still thought this was a mistake. Something which would break her heart when she had risked everything to take a chance on him.

He tucked a strand of her hair behind her ear. 'Now, I think there are a lot more comfortable places than a hard wood table to spend the rest of the day.'

Daisy's heart was beating like a butterfly's wings at all the connotations in that comment. The promise of repeat performances and the prospect of spending the rest of the evening in his bed was all it took for her to abandon her fears about moving in here with him for a while.

This was one time she was willing to give up her independence because it was exactly what she wanted too.

They took some time out to check on the village residents before indulging their erotic fantasies further. Not everyone had been able to salvage their belongings but there seemed little Daisy and Thomas could do for now except patch up those who had sustained minor injuries during the storm.

Selfishly, she couldn't wait to get back to the house to have Thomas to herself. It was admirable that he wished to help everyone as best he could, but they had done their bit and deserved some down time.

'If you need anything at all, call me. We're going to be working out of the house from tomorrow for anyone who needs treatment.' He handed his business card over to one of the locals, making sure everyone knew who to go to for help.

'Are we taking anyone back with us?'

He shook his head. 'A few are going to stay with family and friends, some are booked into hotels and the rest are staying put. It's just us tonight.' He lowered his voice for the last part of his reply, sending shivers of anticipation dancing across the back of Daisy's neck.

'Oh, dear. I hope you're not too upset,' she said, coyly batting her eyelashes at him.

'Not one little bit.' He was looking at her with that fire in his eyes capable of incinerating her on the spot.

'In that case maybe we should—' She tipped her head towards the car.

'Go home? My thoughts exactly.' Thomas made giant strides across to the vehicle, clearly in a hurry.

If it was not for the audience of residents and those Thomas had drafted in to help, Daisy got the impression he would have thrown her over his shoulder and carted her back to his cave.

A completely different person from the superior doctor in the three-piece suit who had looked down his nose at her. Now she knew that was a defence mechanism and self-preservation against people like his ex, she was glad he no longer felt the need to shield from her.

This was the real Thomas Ryan—fun, loyal, passionate and someone she wanted to be around. The sort of bond forming between them was something she had tended to steer clear of, but they were both dealing with similar issues. Venturing into new territory. Though they hadn't discussed where things were going, she was sure they wouldn't want to rush into something serious too soon.

She also thought it wise that they shouldn't engage in any public displays of affection in case the local gossip put them under pressure.

Once they had driven away from the village she leaned her head on Thomas's shoulder. It was nice. Normal. Anyone could be forgiven for thinking they were a regular couple, minus the emotional baggage wedged into the front seat between them.

'I hope you're not falling asleep on me,' he said, dropping a kiss onto her head.

'No. I'm just enjoying the time out from all the drama.' She could easily fall asleep here when she was so content, not to mention worn out by the events of the past few days. Except she didn't want to miss a second of whatever Thomas had planned for tonight. There was no telling how soon this would end so she wanted to make the most of this can't-get-enough-of-one-another phase.

'Don't worry, you can lie back and let me do all the hard work if you're tired.'

'Why, Dr Ryan, are you trying to seduce me?' Daisy knew the second he touched her, her body would be wide awake and raring to go.

'Trying? Obviously I'm not doing a good

enough job of it.' He turned off the engine once they pulled up outside his house, unbuckled his seatbelt and leaned over to undo hers. He was so close she could feel his breath on her cheek. Enough to send arousal rushing through her bloodstream.

Instead of letting the belt retract itself, he slowly drew it up across her chest, deliberately brushing his hand over her breast. Her body ultra-aware of him now, her nipples tightened in response.

'Any better?' he asked, his lips almost touching hers.

'A tad,' she squeaked, waiting with bated breath for him to make a move.

He leaned further across, nuzzling against her neck, and just when she was about to explode with need he reached past her and opened her door.

'Good to see I haven't lost it after all.' The wink he gave her was too much.

'You're in big trouble, mister.' Despite her frustration Daisy was still smiling when she got out of the car. This flirty teasing was exactly what she needed. No stress, no drama, just sexy fun, and this version of Thomas was the man to have it with.

'Good.' Thomas slid his arms around her waist and pulled her roughly to him. Daisy's heart gave that fluttery extra beat it had started doing every time he came near her, the anticipation of his touch sending her pulse and libido into overdrive. Thankfully she didn't have to wait long for her prize.

Thomas bent his head and covered her mouth with his. A leisurely kiss at first, as they took their time exploring one another again, it soon developed into something much more demanding. The lust for one another was too great to be satisfied by one kiss alone. With the knowledge that they had the house to themselves, uninhibited by thoughts of being interrupted, there was no reason to worry about modesty or privacy.

In a frenzy of kissing and undressing, they made their way across the hall. Daisy stumbled back against the stairs, bringing Thomas down with her. Undeterred, he unzipped her trousers and pulled them off, along with everything else until she was lying beneath him in just her bra. Without taking his eyes off her, Thomas stripped off too.

Daisy watched him, her chest rising and falling with every shallow breath she took. This had to be one of the most erotic moments of her life, but it was also one of the most uncomfortable.

'Thomas?'

'Yes?' He was kissing her neck, his body on top of hers, his erection pressing between her thighs. She was wet and ready for him, but not here with the edges of the stairs bruising her back.

'I thought we were going to do this somewhere more comfortable this time?'

Thomas laughed and levered himself up off her. 'You're right. My bad.'

He offered his hand and helped her to her feet. 'Bedroom. Now.'

Giggling, Daisy took off towards his room with him chasing her. They were acting like two hormonal teenagers in the first throes of passion, but that was what was making this so easy for her. She didn't have to think when her body was doing the talking for her. When she and Thomas were having fun she could forget the serious stuff. There was no need to overthink things like what would happen between them at work or the prospect of giving up her independence to start a relationship with another man. For now, this was just sex and that suited her fine.

Thomas caught up with her, grabbing her waist from behind and making her squeal. It was thrilling to be in the house alone, making as much noise as they dared and not caring about anything other than reaching that big comfortable bed. Here they were both free from the shackles of the past and at liberty to revel in their sensuality.

As if to prove the point, Thomas unfastened her bra and let it fall to the floor, taking the weight of her breasts in his hands. He teased the peaks between his fingers and that, combined with his hot breath at her ear and his hardness pressed against her buttocks, meant Daisy was a puddle of arousal. She spun around to kiss him and pulled him down onto the bed.

'I want you, Thomas.' She was begging him to fulfil that aching need for him but, instead of covering her body with his, he lay down beside her.

'Soon,' he said and kissed her on the lips. He grabbed a condom from the bedside table and rolled it down over his erection, Daisy watching his every move with anticipation.

She turned onto her side, pressing herself against him, desperate for that ultimate connection between them. He took her breast in his hand and ran his tongue over the mound, teasing her nipple until it stood proud. The sharp tug of his mouth as he sucked was pleasant torture and she closed her eyes to let the sensation wash over her.

Thomas slipped his hand down between

their bodies and dipped his fingers into her very core.

'You're so wet,' he growled, his voice filled with undisguised lust.

Daisy was so wrapped up in what he was doing to her she couldn't find the words to respond. With masterful fingers he massaged and stroked the most sensitive part of her until he had her bucking off the bed with pure want. Her breathing was rapid as the pressure built up inside her. She clutched at his chest, desperate for something to hold on to as she soared away on that feeling of bliss. It pushed him to delve deeper, faster, hastening her climax. It overwhelmed her both physically and mentally that he could do this to her so easily. Commanding her body with so little effort made her fear that she was losing control. The warning flashing in the distance disturbing her euphoria brought her abruptly back to earth. She pushed Thomas's hand away.

'Is something wrong? Did I hurt you?'

'No. I'm simply taking the initiative.' Daisy moved across to straddle his hips, taking charge again.

'Oh, yes? I thought we agreed I was going to do all the hard work tonight?' He was grinning from ear to ear, content about the shift in power. An aphrodisiac in itself if she had needed it.

'I'm all for equal rights,' she said, sliding her body along his length to make them both groan with need.

'Me too,' he gasped, taking a possessive hold of her wrist as she bore down onto his erection. She was temporarily stunned into silence as he filled her but that need to make a snarky comeback was obliterated by the need to have all of Thomas. To render him speechless, his body at her mercy this time.

Daisy rocked her hips back and forth, bracing herself with a hand on his chest. He was watching her intently as she used his body to pleasure herself. All the time she held his gaze, increasing the pace and stoking the fire within.

Thomas shifted into a sitting position, grabbing the back of her head and kissing her, distracting her from other parts of his body using his mouth and tongue. That control was slipping, that focus on keeping this about sex when he was kissing her so tenderly and trying to make her feel something more than physical need.

She pushed him back down, slid up and down his shaft with renewed determination. Thomas cried out and she grinned, knowing she had got the upper hand again. Then he grabbed her hips and thrust upwards, surprising her into a gasp of ecstasy. They moved together now, both striving to find their ultimate satisfaction. Daisy realised it was better when they were in sync, each wanting to please the other, caring about their partner's needs as well as their own. Somewhere deep inside she knew it meant something, but she was too consumed by this race to bring their release to care.

She didn't even mind when Thomas somehow ended up on top again, manoeuvring her legs over his shoulders so he could plunge deeper inside her. Daisy closed her eyes, gave herself over to the things he was making her feel. Stopped fighting it. When her orgasm came, her eyes were wet with tears.

Thomas couldn't hold back any longer when she was calling out his name with her climax, squeezing him tight as she came. Daisy did things to him he couldn't explain—and didn't want to examine too closely. So far they had been keeping things light, not daring to venture beyond the amazing sex and good times together. As though they were afraid that whatever it was when acknowledged would burst the bubble and remind them that they had to deal with the real world.

Yet when they were lying in bed together, trying desperately to catch their breath, bodies glowing from their exertions, he wanted a deeper connection that went beyond the bedroom door or the kitchen table.

He rolled onto his side and watched her smiling through those panting breaths she was trying to regulate. Daisy was beautiful, sexy and fun and everything he had been missing in his life. He didn't know what he was afraid of any more. She wasn't his ex, she wasn't going to betray him when they were working and living together, albeit temporary. Perhaps it was time he stopped punishing himself for things he hadn't done. Started living life to the full instead of hiding away, afraid of getting hurt. He needed to be honest about what he felt for Daisy.

With a sudden rush of blood to his head, he wanted to share this revelation with her. Tell her how much she had done to help him get to this point and how he felt about her. He was falling for her, beginning to think they could have a future together if only they could move past the reservations they both had about committing to anyone again.

'Daisy, I—'

'Shh.' She put her finger on his lips. Whatever he might have been going to say, obviously she wasn't ready to hear it.

CHAPTER NINE

THOMAS LEFT DAISY sleeping to get a head start on the day. He'd been thinking about the evolution of their relationship, what it meant to him and how they were going to proceed. Following his old pattern, he should draw a line under what had happened between them and halt any progression. He'd been wary of women and relationships in general because of his mother's actions and Jade had only cemented that belief that he couldn't trust anyone, that it would only lead to heartbreak.

Daisy was making him reconsider that belief. At least to the point where he was willing to take a chance that things could be different. He thought they could have a real chance of something special when they had already pushed through some of their fears to be together. She had given him the impetus to want to make changes in his life because he wanted her in it. If only she felt the same.

When she had so many scars from the past yet to heal, Thomas was aware that taking the next step into a proper relationship would be a big deal for her. He wanted her to feel safe, to know that he was willing to share everything he had and take that risk to his heart and his home if he could be with her.

Thomas set to work making arrangements so that Daisy would know he was serious about her. They had already talked about working out of his house until the clinic was safe again, so he organised that while she slept. It was no wonder she was exhausted after everything she had been through these past few days, so he let her sleep while he set up her office in one of the front rooms. He cleared away the ugly antiques, garish statues and drab paintings he'd lived with as a tribute to his father and put them into storage. In an effort to make Daisy more at ease so she could treat this as her own space, he dotted her things around. The houseplant someone had given her as a gift, the knick-knacks and stationery he had rescued from her desk and the London cityscape she'd had hanging on her wall now adorned the walls of her new office.

It was his way of telling her she was part of his life and he welcomed that development rather than fearing it.

They still had a long way to go. Thomas couldn't say what would happen long-term between them. He wasn't sure if he would ever find the courage to completely open up his heart and his life to the point of marriage or children. There was no way of knowing if Daisy would even want that, but this was a gesture to tell her he was willing to begin that journey with her. That he trusted her enough to try.

'What is going on?' Some time later Daisy wandered into the room he had allocated as his office. His last patient had just left so he was filling in some notes when she walked in.

'Morning. I opened the clinic early for walk-in patients but now you're here we can split the list between us.'

'That explains all the coming and going. I thought I was imagining it.' She yawned and took a sip from the cup of tea sitting on his desk.

'Take it. Eunice keeps making tea for everyone to keep herself busy.' He pushed the cup back towards her, knowing she needed that first cup before she started her day.

Daisy wrapped her hands around the cup and breathed in the steam. 'Eunice is here too?'

'I've set up a waiting area with her desk in

it so she can point people in the right direction. It's not an ideal set-up but hopefully it won't be for long.'

'In that case, I suppose I should get started. Where should I go?'

'I've allocated you the other front room for your office. If there are any problems just let me know.'

'I will need to swing by the cottage to get some more of my work clothes and toiletries to see me through.'

'No problem. Although it's going to take a while for the cottage to dry out, never mind the time it will take to get the place redecorated and furnished. You're going to need to bring most of your personal things.'

'It would probably be easier for me to just move in,' she joked, but Thomas didn't think that was a bad idea at all when she was living with him anyway.

'Right, I must go and get ready to face the day. Thanks for the tea.' Daisy raised the cup before she walked away. It wasn't the warm reunion he might have been hoping for, but she was likely trying to process last night's events too.

Thomas would do everything he could to make Daisy comfortable in his home and she had given him the perfect idea. Once she saw the lengths he was willing to go to in order to welcome her into his life, he was convinced any wariness she had around their current situation would soon evaporate. This was going to be the start of something great between them.

There was something about having the contents of her office suddenly appear here which unnerved Daisy. She knew Thomas had only been trying to make her feel comfortable, but she wasn't used to people doing things for her. It automatically put her on edge. Invariably when her ex, or even her stepfather, had done anything remotely nice for her, there was usually a motive behind it. In the case of her stepfamily, they used to humiliate her afterwards.

Like the time when her stepfather had built up her hopes for weeks, telling her he had got her something special for Christmas, something no one else would have. At ten years old she had believed him, and told all her friends about this amazing present she was getting. Only to unwrap a chocolate Easter egg on Christmas morning, her disappointment caught on camera and shared as a source of amusement, making a laughing stock of her.

It was not by any means the cruellest stunt pulled on her but one which had stuck in her mind. Mostly because her stepfather had let her believe that he genuinely cared, that she was special and that life might be getting better for her. Only to receive expired chocolate while her stepbrothers enjoyed the latest games console, which she wasn't allowed to touch.

Then there was her ex. Aaron would buy her gifts to make her feel indebted to him. If she wanted to see her friends or do anything with anyone other than him she was met with sad eyes and, 'No one loves you the way I love you. Who else buys you the things I buy you? No one. You don't need anyone but me.'

Of course there were also the gifts after he had lashed out at her in temper. Flowers and chocolates to make her forget about the cuts and bruises.

Thomas was neither of those men who had emotionally abused her for their own agendas, but it was difficult to change her mindset after all this time of living on her own. In order to protect herself she had learned to be wary. She was still afraid that he might be doing these things for her in a subconscious attempt to control her. He had made it known he had issues with trust, and she could understand to some extent that he had a need to take charge to prevent himself getting hurt. However, she was not prepared to lose herself simply so that he could feel protected.

It was likely that all they needed was a conversation to explain her need for some space without offending him. He had a kind heart. She had seen that for herself. And it wasn't his fault that she felt unable to reap the benefits of that. Nevertheless, that feeling of needing to protect herself was valid and there for a reason—so she didn't end up in the same predicament she had been in with her first serious relationship. If she and Thomas decided this was going to become more than sleeping together he would have to understand her need to take things slowly.

Although they had made love again last night Daisy had slept in the spare room, telling him she needed a full night's sleep and wouldn't get that if they were in the same bed. It was partly true. She had also needed a bit of space to herself. The early days of a new relationship were a challenge for her, and she didn't want to seem ungrateful when Thomas was simply trying to help her adapt to the new surroundings. Even if she found it a tad overwhelming so soon.

It was plausible that the nerves she had

about getting into a relationship had caused her to catastrophize when he had only hoped to put her at ease. That she was projecting her issues from the past when he had made a loving gesture to show her he was ready to share his living space.

At least Daisy had her patients to fill her day and the sense of uneasiness she initially experienced seeing her new temporary office gradually subsided.

'I will chase up that consultant appointment for you at the hospital, Mrs Cooper, and in the meantime I'll continue to see you every couple of weeks.' Daisy stood up to see her patient out and wished as she always did in these cases that waiting lists for hospital treatment were not so long.

The elderly woman took some time to get across the floor on her walking stick. Daisy had done everything she could to relieve the pain in her knees, but she really needed surgery to make any long-term difference. 'Thank you, Dr Swift. I'm so glad you and Dr Ryan are still able to see patients.'

'So am I,' Daisy said, and she meant it. She needed some sense of normality, to be in her comfort zone, when things around her seemed to be out of her control.

Her libido in particular, whenever she happened to see Thomas. He was at the door of his office saying goodbye to his patient too. She took her chance to satisfy her thirst for him.

'Dr Ryan, could I see you in your office for a moment, please?'

'Sure—'

She barely gave Thomas the time to answer before she pushed him back through the door, kicking it shut behind her. It didn't take him long to get with the programme, taking her face in his hands and kissing her passionately on the lips. Daisy nearly slid down onto the floor in a puddle of arousal and would have let him take her there and then if Eunice hadn't buzzed through on the intercom.

'Dr Ryan, your next patient is here to see you.'

Thomas slowly peeled away from her, a smile on his lips now instead of her. 'No rest for the wicked.'

'I guess not,' she said, wiping the smudges of lipstick she was sure were round her mouth, giving away exactly what they had been up to.

'Can we pick this up later, after work?'

'Of course, Dr Ryan. I am here at your disposal,' she said with a coy wink, putting any doubts about what was going on between them behind her for now to enjoy the flirtation.

It wasn't Thomas's fault she had been displaced from her house. He hadn't arranged a devastating flood just so he could get her under his roof. No, he had offered her a place to stay, regardless that up until the night of the storm he had been reluctant to let anyone cross his threshold. He had done his best to make her feel comfortable. She should be grateful to Thomas for his kindness. Everyone else in the village was certainly enamoured with him. Any time she saw him with one of the residents, they were enthusiastically shaking his hand or slapping him on the back, thanking him for all of his help. Now that she and Thomas had taken the next step in their relationship, it would be a shame for her paranoia to creep in and ruin everything.

Daisy made the decision there and then to simply enjoy being with Thomas and not to let the past steal away her future.

It was crazy to think of his family home being used as a makeshift surgery, but there was also something incredibly natural about winding down with Daisy after work. With the staff and patients gone, this was their time and Thomas had been looking forward to it all day. Along with more of those delicious kisses they stole any time they had a break in their schedule.

'Dinner?' he asked as she kicked off her heels at the front door once they had waved Eunice off for the night.

'Yes, please, but can we have something here? I don't really feel like going out.' She wrapped her arms around him and planted a leisurely kiss on his mouth.

It was nice not to be facing a night alone with nothing but the TV and paperwork to keep him company.

'No problem. I'm sure I can fix us something to eat. I'll see what we've got in the fridge.'

'You cook?' Daisy's incredulity was evident as she followed him through to the kitchen.

He laughed as he set to work making dinner for two, a novelty for him since losing his father. 'I'm a grown man. Yes, I can cook.'

'I just assumed you would order in or, you know, have your own private chef on call twenty-four hours a day.'

Thomas rolled his eyes as he passed the

contents of his fridge to Daisy to set on the kitchen worktop.

'I like to cook. I haven't done much of it since Dad died. This makes a nice change.' He held up a bottle of white wine and Daisy nodded her approval.

'For me too. I can't remember the last time anyone cooked for me.' Daisy was about to make herself comfortable when Thomas poured two glasses of wine and put some mood music on in the background. He wanted her to feel more at home than simply a dinner guest.

'Who said I was doing all of the cooking? You can be my sous chef.' He pushed a chopping board and knife towards her, along with some garlic and vegetables.

Daisy let out an exaggerated sigh before setting to work chopping the ingredients.

'I hope a stir-fry is okay for you?' Thomas diced some chicken and added it to the hot pan on the stove. Once it was seared, he added the vegetables, some soy sauce and chilli and tossed in some noodles.

'Definitely. I'm starving.'

Thomas dished up the meal while Daisy carried their glasses of wine to the table. It was nice, normal, to be making dinner as a couple, looking forward to spending the rest of the night chilling out together. A routine he could get used to quite easily.

'Here's to us,' he said, raising his glass to hers. 'We make a good team.'

Daisy was smiling as she joined the toast. 'And a good stir-fry, apparently.'

They ate in companionable silence, content to fill their bellies and simply enjoy winding down from their working day. Thomas went to top up the wine glasses, but Daisy covered hers with a hand.

'I've had enough. If you don't mind I'd like to go to bed.' She got up from her chair and left her dishes in the sink.

'No problem.' He knew all the upheaval had probably exhausted her and it would be selfish of him to ask her to stay with him merely because he wanted more of her company.

She moved to the kitchen door and glanced back, her hand outstretched towards him. 'Aren't you coming?'

Thomas almost kicked over the table in his haste to join her. When Daisy was taking him to bed he knew it would involve more than sleep. That was something she apparently preferred to do on her own, and though he would prefer to wake up next to her in the mornings he was prepared to wait until she was ready to share his bed all night. Whatever it took for her to be comfortable and remain in his life. Daisy was one habit he didn't want to break.

CHAPTER TEN

'Wakey-wakey.'

Daisy was shaken from her slumber by the sound of Thomas's voice and a hand on her arm.

'What time is it?' she mumbled into her pillow, her eyes and body refusing to wake.

'Early.'

'I thought so,' she said and rolled over to get comfortable again.

The rustle of the sheets and a sudden blast of cold air on her skin told her he wasn't taking no for an answer as he pulled away her covers. She groaned. She was not a morning person.

'Come on. I have something planned for us.' He sounded like an excited little kid, which at any other time of the day she would think was adorable.

'What?' She still refused to move her face out of her pillow to look at him. It would have to be something pretty special to make her want to leave this bed if she didn't have to.

'Look,' he coaxed.

When she didn't move he kissed her cheek. That wasn't playing fair when he knew she couldn't resist his touch. Daisy brushed her hair from her eyes and squinted over at him. 'What is it?'

He was holding up something black and wearing what seemed like a skin-tight all-in-one. She blinked furiously, trying to focus so she could see what on earth he was trying to get her to do.

'It's a wetsuit. I've already got mine on.'

'Ugh.' She collapsed back into her feather haven when he failed to convince her there was somewhere better to be than here. It definitely was not in freezing-cold water making a fool of herself doing whatever it was Thomas had in mind.

'You helped me face my fears by inviting people into my home, now I want to help you tackle one of yours. Put this on and meet me down by the harbour.' The wetsuit landed on top of her and Thomas left the room, apparently confident that she would acquiesce to his demands and go to him rather than leave him standing there waiting. He was right.

She knew he was only trying to do something nice for her and since he had set aside his fears when she'd asked him it was time she did the same. She was afraid of the water because she couldn't swim but she was certain Thomas wasn't about to let her drown. It would take a lot of trust on her part, but that was an important element in a relationship. If they were ever going to make it she had to learn to have faith in him. After all, he had proved his worth these past weeks, to her and the rest of the community.

With a lot of puffing, panting and swearing, Daisy wriggled her way into the tight costume, knowing her reward would be seeing Thomas in his. She hadn't taken the chance to ogle him properly, but that would soon be rectified now she was awake and missing his presence in the bedroom. If she did this for him, showed willing, maybe she could persuade him to come back for an afternoon nap…

If she'd gone with Thomas when he'd asked, there would have been no need for her to take her car down to the harbour too. It seemed scandalous to be driving to the village wearing so little, yet it was acceptable dress around here with the locals and their love of water sports. Still, she opened the barrier and drove down to the harbour rather than parade through the streets in her figure-hugging outfit which left nothing to the imagination.

The village was slowly getting back to normal, though most days the air was filled with dust and noise as builders and carpenters set to work repairing that which had been lost or ruined in the flood. Given the early hour of the morning, though, everything was quiet now. Everyone but her apparently had the luxury of sleeping in on a Saturday morning. She couldn't complain, not really. These past couple of weeks with Thomas hadn't been a hardship. They worked together, relaxed over a bottle of wine as they made dinner at night and made love before they went their separate ways to sleep. It was a life she could easily get used to.

This morning was out of the norm from their usual routine but at least she had the sight of Thomas, bare-chested, his wetsuit hanging open to his waist, all to herself. He was walking across the small strip of the sandy shore at the harbour's edge with two large boards under his arms. Daisy groaned as she parked the car and got out to join him, knowing this was the last time she was going to be safe on dry land for a while. What was it about this man and water?

'Morning,' she said, enjoying the view of her gorgeous man coming towards her, so happy to see her he had broken into a run.

'Morning.' He grabbed her around the waist and swung her around and kissed her on her lips.

'That's some welcome.' She was breathless and giddy and unsure why she had wanted any time apart from him when she felt so good in his arms.

'You're in better form too, I see. I didn't realise you were so grumpy in the morning.' His teasing earned him a playful slap on the arm.

'Only when people wake me up at a ridiculous hour with the sole intention of trying to drown me.' She glanced at the boards. Surfing? Surely he was not expecting her to be comfortable with that? Trepidation crept in and she suddenly wondered why she thought keeping Thomas satisfied was better than keeping herself safe. Surely that was the old way of thinking which had got her into trouble before?

Before she could worry herself into a state, Thomas started to laugh.

'I assure you what I have planned is nothing as dangerous or dramatic as that. I thought it would be good for us to get out and do something that didn't revolve around work. Have fun. Remember that?' That twinkle in his eye was just as alluring as the unzipped wetsuit just waiting to be stripped all the way off his body.

'What have you got planned?' She sighed, resolved to do whatever it was he was so keen for her to take part in.

'Paddleboarding.'

'Paddleboarding?' she repeated. 'What if something takes a huge chunk out of me or I fall off and drown?'

'We'll be doing it in the harbour, where nothing is going to bite you and you will be wearing one of these.' He let go of her and reached for one of the lifejackets laid out on the sand.

'In the harbour where there are millions of pounds' worth of yachts I can crash into,' she huffed as she donned the bulky buoyancy aid.

Thomas zipped up his wetsuit and put his on too. 'You are not going to crash into anything, drown or get eaten by a shark. The point is to have fun and learn something new. Now, no more excuses. Get on your board.'

Daisy eyed him with suspicion. 'Here? How exactly are we going to paddle on the sand?'

He resisted rising to her sarcasm and passed

her a paddle. 'I'm giving you your first lesson before we get in the water. Trust me, you'll thank me for it.'

Daisy doubted it. Nothing about this was her idea of fun, except for the fantasy of peeling that rubber suit off him later. Only then might she be grateful to him for suggesting they do this.

'I'm on the board, I've got my paddle—now what?'

'Get on your knees.'

'Ooh, Dr Ryan, you're so masterful.' If he wanted her to have fun he had to expect some teasing on her part too. Especially when they could be enjoying each other's company back in the comfort of a bed.

'You need to start off on your knees so you can get your balance right.' He demonstrated the move without acknowledging her childish innuendo. In the end she gave up fighting his attempt to teach her how to paddleboard and literally got on board.

'Okay, so I'm on my knees. Now what?'

'That lowers your centre of gravity so you can stabilise yourself. Once you're comfortable enough to take the next step, place your oar across the board, move up onto one foot and then the other so you're in a squatting position.'

'I think I can manage that.' She watched Thomas do it first and though the moves were easy enough to emulate now she knew it would be a different story when she was out there on the water.

'If you keep looking out across the water instead of looking at your feet it will help you centre your balance as you stand up.'

'What happens if I overbalance and fall off?'

'You get back on. Your board will be tethered to your ankle so it won't float away from you.' Thomas went on to show her the basic strokes she would need to get her board moving and how to use the paddle to turn her around.

'Is that the first lesson over? Can we go home now?' she asked, dreading what was coming next and praying he would show some mercy. No chance.

'This is just the start. All the fun is still to come.' He was grinning as he picked up his board and walked towards the water, beckoning her to come with him.

'I wouldn't do this for anyone else, you know,' she grumbled, joining him in the shallows.

'And I appreciate it. I might just forget about the dunk tank incident after this.' He reminded her he had done a lot to keep her happy over these last weeks and now it was her turn she didn't want to disappoint.

'Okay, now, how do I get on without toppling the whole thing over?' Daisy was looking at it like a hammock scenario where the wrong distribution of weight could see her capsized and flailing about like a helpless turtle on its back.

'Get on it here where it's not too deep and paddle your way out. Don't worry, I'll be beside you all the way.' True to his word, Thomas waded out with her as she managed to get onto her board and on her knees and made her way further out into the harbour.

This was all new for her. It was terrifying and exhilarating that she was facing one of her fears without overanalysing the possible outcome. A process she should apply to her other issues if she ever hoped to move on. She had taken that first step by accepting Thomas was here to stay in her life but making that next risky move would take all of her courage. It was the fear of being left floundering on her own which prevented her from trying.

Thomas jumped athletically onto his board and paddled out alongside her. 'See? Easypeasy. Now, when you're ready, try and get up onto your feet.'

She wondered why she couldn't just coast along like this, where she was comfortable, but Thomas would only tell her she was missing out on so much more. A metaphor for her entire life. It gave her the impetus to strike out and take a risk for once in her life and damn the consequences. What was life if she didn't experience new adventures once in a while?

Very slowly, she unfurled one leg from beneath her. It had started to go to sleep so it was better she did it now before her entire lower half was numb and she toppled into the harbour like a drunken sailor on shore leave.

'That's it. Keep looking ahead and get that other foot up there too.' Thomas called his encouragement to her, but she was too busy trying not to look at her feet to spare him a glance or nod.

The second foot was much trickier.

'Woah!' The board was wobbling about under her as she attempted to master that sit-down crouch which was so much easier on dry land. Everything went into slow motion as she tried to stop the inevitable. Try as she might, she couldn't get her balance and she felt herself falling into the abyss.

The water went in her mouth and up her nose, leaving her gasping for breath. She was splashing around in distress even though common sense told her she was wearing a life jacket and close to shore.

'You're okay. I've got you.' Thomas's calm voice broke through her panic as he jumped into the water beside her.

'I told you, I can't do this,' she blubbed, hoping no one else was watching her epic fail. It was bad enough Thomas had witnessed it and she probably looked like something that had been washed ashore in a storm with her wet hair and mascara-stained face.

'Yes, you can. It wasn't long ago you were underwater helping to rescue old Jimmy. I'm sure you're not going to let a paddleboard beat you.' Thomas appealed to that stubborn streak inside her and he was right. She had held it together through all their trials during the storm, at least until she had seen her own place, so a stupid lump of fibreglass wasn't going to defeat her. It wasn't the end of the world because she had fallen into the water; she was still alive and still spending the morning with this lovely man.

'Well, give us a hand up then,' she said, wiping the water from her eyes and grabbing her paddle before it drifted too far away from her.

'Yes, ma'am.' Thomas obliged with a helping hand on her posterior as she clambered back onto her board in a more ungainly fashion than she had first time around.

'Okay, let's do this,' she whispered to herself before she could overthink things and chicken out. One foot. Two feet. She wobbled but managed to steady herself again and very carefully stood up from her crouching position. It was tempting to cheer or punch the air in celebration, but she didn't want to risk toppling over again. Thomas did it for her.

'Woo-hoo! Go, Daisy!' He slapped the surface of the water with the flat of his hand, sending a celebratory shower over her.

'Thomas! Careful before you knock me off-balance again!' She fought to stay upright as the board rocked against the motion of the disturbed water. Though this time the thought of falling in again wasn't nearly as terrifying. It hadn't killed her, only wrecked her hair. Even if she did get into trouble, she trusted Thomas to save her.

If only she could find the same courage to believe in them as a couple they might have a future together. That meant she would have to stop overthinking all the different ways she could end up getting hurt and show the same trust in Thomas as a partner as she did in him as an instructor.

* * *

Thomas was pleased he'd been able to convince Daisy to come down here this morning. He'd left the decision entirely up to her, not wishing to push her too far when he knew how difficult it was to face one's fears. If it had not been for the flood, his neighbours' distress and Daisy's nudging, he might never have invited another living soul back into the family home. He was glad he had, as now it seemed as though the gloom had lifted from the house so the sun shone in every corner once more. All he wanted for Daisy was that same freedom. To release her from whatever pain she still held from the past to enjoy every day fully.

Thank goodness the paddleboarding had turned out to be a good idea. That early fall had made his heart stop and his breath catch, fearing that it would trigger whatever trauma continued to wreak havoc in Daisy about the water. He should have known her bravery would win through and she would push herself to the limit, as she had done since she'd first arrived in Little Morton.

Indeed, they had both fallen into the water a few times during their lesson, but now they were coasting contentedly around the harbour. Daisy was no longer frowning in concentration trying to maintain her balance but smiling and enjoying the feel of the sun on her face.

'Thank you for doing this, Daisy.' Thomas was aware she had only agreed to come here because he had asked her to. It meant the world to him, not only that she had got out of bed for him but because she had confronted her fear simply so they could spend more time together. The fact that they were both willing to make sacrifices for one another was a good omen for their blossoming relationship.

Until recently he had thought himself incapable of feeling anything other than fear and distrust, doing little more than going through the motions of daily life. With Daisy there was genuine affection, passion and longing running through his veins again like electricity, sparking his body back to life and giving him something to look forward to every day. Being with her had given him a new lease of life. He didn't know what he had to offer her in return, but he hoped this was a start. They both needed a little time out just to chill and enjoy each other's company like this. Hopefully it would become a regular occurrence.

'I'm actually glad I came. There's something peaceful about skimming across the water with no one else around. I can see why you wanted to do this so early in the morning. You can't hear anything except the seagulls and the boats bobbing around us.' Daisy looked so at peace in the surroundings it seemed the perfect antidote to the stress and drama working at the clinic often brought. That was why he had taken up paddleboarding himself. Although he had rented Daisy's wetsuit and board, he had his own. He wasn't a surfer or someone who got his kicks on high-powered jet skis and speedboats. This got him out of the house and gave him all the benefits of the fresh sea air without risking any serious injury which could put him out of action at work for any length of time. Now it seemed like something they could do as a couple, with the added bonus of seeing Daisy in skin-tight fabric.

Even with her hair wet and devoid of her usual swipe of red lipstick, he couldn't wait to get his hands on her again. This wasn't like it had been with Jade, when he'd rushed blindly into a relationship without knowing what he was getting into. He and Daisy had fought against this attraction from the start. They had shared a lot about their pasts and the residual issues they harboured as a result. He had agonised over the consequences of them being together, yet he wanted her more than he had ever wanted anyone or anything in his life before. There seemed little point in wasting any more time when he was certain Daisy was the one he was willing to risk everything for.

'And no one to see what we get up to,' he said, moving until his board was parallel with hers.

'What are you doing?' she asked, eyebrows raised as she watched him set down his paddle and set one foot onto her board.

'I have gone too long without kissing you and I need to rectify that.' Once he had himself balanced between the two boards, he made the leap across so he was facing Daisy.

'You're mad!'

He grabbed hold of her and kissed her long and hard as the paddleboard shifted beneath them with his added weight. They were still clinging to one another when they overbalanced and plunged into the water.

Thomas couldn't have been more apologetic when Daisy came spluttering back to the surface. 'I'm so sorry. I didn't mean... I'm such an idiot... I was only trying to... Sorry, Daisy.'

He pulled her board over and held it steady until she was back upright and, thankfully, still smiling.

'It's good to know I'm so irresistible, but perhaps we should take this back onto dry land, lover boy.' When she blew him a kiss and headed back to shore Thomas wasted no time in paddling after her. They had enjoyed their early morning leisure pursuit and put a few demons to rest in the process. There was enough time for them to have a little more fun back home before they were needed else-where.

Back on the beach, he untethered his board and went to Daisy so they could pick up where they had left off without the unexpected cold bath. Her lips tasted like the sea, her little sat-isfied groans like a siren's call, and he would have willingly gone to his death for just one more kiss.

'What if someone see us?' she asked with-out any real urgency.

'I don't care.' It was the truth. They were both young and single; what they did in their private lives was no one else's concern. He'd been using the possibility of village gossip damaging his reputation as another excuse to avoid getting hurt. Rather than being afraid of people knowing they were together, he'd been more concerned about what he thought would be an inevitable break-up in the spot-light. He'd had no desire to suffer his next heartbreak in front of an audience. Now, though, he was doing his best to be as brave as Daisy had shown herself to be today and throw himself into this at full pelt. It seemed as though they were both ready to start living again and he, for one, was looking forward to all the surprises that would bring.

'It's just as well. I think that's Eunice over there walking her dog.'

Thomas instantly moved out of the embrace to see what Daisy was talking about. Sure enough, his trusty receptionist was up along the promenade with her dachshund tottering alongside her. If she saw them together the whole village would know by lunchtime. His personal life didn't come under the confidentiality clause in her contract.

In an act of bravado or defiance against those who had caused him pain in the past, Thomas pulled Daisy close to him. He bent her back and planted a Hollywood-style kiss on her mouth so there would be no mistaking what was going on between them.

Beyond the sound of blood pounding in his ears he heard clapping and whistling, followed by the sound of Eunice's voice. 'It's about damned time.'

He leaned his forehead against Daisy's. 'I hope that was okay with you?'

She nodded and gave him another peck on the lips in return, gaining another round of applause from Eunice. A chorus of whoops went up as others had apparently gathered with their receptionist to witness their very public display of affection.

'I guess there's no going back now,' Daisy said, sounding every bit as nervous as Thomas felt.

Daisy was guilty of daydreaming in between appointments. Letting her thoughts drift to the previous night and the incredible time she'd had in bed with Thomas was becoming a habit. At times she even found herself loitering in the hall, waiting to catch a glimpse of him or, if she was really lucky, grab him for a quick kiss. Man, she had it bad.

When it came to the end of another day's surgery, she was bursting to spend some quality time with Thomas.

'See you tomorrow, Eunice.' She waved the receptionist off at the front door, then closed and locked it.

'Has everyone gone now?' Thomas came up behind her, his arms sliding effortlessly around her waist. Daisy leaned back against him, the tension of the day leaving her body to let arousal take its place.

'Yes.' She couldn't wait any longer to take her fill of him, kissing him as though she hadn't seen him for months instead of hours.

'Do you want to get some dinner or—?' He didn't have to say what else he was thinking about when Daisy's mind was already racing upstairs with him.

'Or?' she said, taking him by the hand to catch up with their runaway thoughts.

'We can get takeaway later if you like? When you see what I have for you upstairs you're not going to want to leave.'

'Promises, promises.' She grinned, hurrying up the stairs hand in hand with Thomas, eager to see just what he had in store for her.

Nothing could have prepared her for what he had done. Instead of taking her into his room, he led her to the room next door. 'I know you like having your own space. Although I'm hoping you'll be spending most nights in my bed.'

Daisy wasn't listening to him. She was too gobsmacked by what she was seeing. 'What have you done, Thomas?'

While she hovered at the door, unsure whether to stay or run, Thomas walked into the room and opened the wardrobe door to show her all of her clothes hanging on the rail. *All* of her clothes. Not just the ones she had packed herself.

That was as unsettling as seeing all of her perfume, make-up and jewellery laid out on top of the mirrored dressing table.

'I thought it would be easier for you to have your stuff here so you didn't have to go back and forward to the cottage.' Clearly oblivious to her discomfort, Thomas continued to show her all of her transferred belongings. He had moved her in without even asking if that was something she wanted. It wasn't.

Red flags were waving everywhere. She hadn't been consulted on something as huge as living with him on a more permanent basis and that absolutely freaked her out. It was too much too soon and making her feel suffocated. All those old feelings came rushing in, overwhelming her with thoughts of what this could be leading to. This was how her ex had started out, with little gestures she'd thought were sweet, until she'd realised he had manipulated her, cut her off from everyone else and any sort of independence. With this move, Thomas was making sure he was becoming her whole world when they would be with each other twenty-four hours a day. Even if his motive was altruistic, she couldn't take the chance of falling into that same trap, thinking she had to do whatever it took to make him happy if she was living in his house and working in his practice, with nowhere else to turn.

'I never said I wanted this.'

'It was you who mentioned things would be easier if you just moved in. I thought it would be a nice surprise.' His smile was beginning to falter as Daisy made it clear she wasn't happy about the situation he had forced her into.

'I wasn't being serious. Why on earth would you think I would want you to move my things in without my permission?' She opened one of the neatly stacked boxes to find the rest of her clothes all folded inside. The other boxes were labelled with 'Toiletries', 'Shoes', and 'Underwear'. Her shudder was probably not the response he had anticipated, but it was such an intrusion into her life she didn't think she would ever get over it.

'I got professional movers in. They were all women and very respectful of your belongings,' Thomas explained, as though that made the slightest bit of difference to her.

'I don't care. You had no right to do this.' Her skin was hot and clammy, her pulse racing so fast it was making her nauseated. She had to get away from here and fast.

'Okay, I got it wrong, but don't you think you're overreacting the tiniest bit, Daisy? This wasn't some attempt to take over your life. I was simply trying to make things easier for you.'

He had absolutely no right to be offended by her reaction when he was the one in the wrong. If he had stopped to think about her, what she had fought against in the past, he would have realised this was the last thing she would have wanted. No, Thomas had only been thinking about what he wanted. Now he was over his people phobia he thought he could move her in here for the sake of convenience and expect her to go along with it because he was her boss as well as her landlord.

'No, I don't think I'm overreacting. We might be sleeping together but that certainly doesn't make you entitled to go onto my property and mess with my things.' If he wanted to be particularly facetious he could point out it was his property and as landlord he did have rights to enter the property, but Daisy was counting on him knowing better than to contradict her in the heat of the moment.

'I wasn't trying to force you into anything. It could just be a temporary arrangement until everything gets back to normal.'

'You had no right.' Her fists were bunched

at her sides, an involuntary action as she got ready to fight for her independence. Flashbacks were terrorising her with images of her ex locking the front door and refusing to give her a key because she didn't need to go anywhere without him.

'I want everything put back now or, better still, I'll take it myself.' She began collecting her bits and pieces, even though she couldn't possibly carry everything herself, but she wasn't thinking clearly. How could she when her past life was flashing before her eyes?

'I'm sorry, Daisy. I didn't mean to upset you, but it's done now.' Thomas moved and took the large can of hairspray from her, which she was trying to shove into her pocket without success.

It was happening. He was undermining her, taking away her freedom, not even allowing her to think or speak for herself without being ridiculed. She was done. There was no way she was putting herself back in this situation.

'Yes, it is, and so are we, Thomas. I should have listened to my instincts from the start. This was never going to work. I can't be here any more. I can't be with you.' Daisy turned on her heel so she could get out as soon as possible. With Thomas's reluctance to take her fears seriously she was feeling more trapped than ever.

'Can't we talk about this?'

'Apparently not. I'll stay somewhere else tonight. The cottage, the pub, wherever…but I will not spend another night here. Don't worry, I'll show up for work. At least until I can find a position elsewhere. I should never have come.' She walked away, shaking her head and cursing herself for repeating past mistakes. Letting her guard down had only left the door open for someone else who thought he could take over her life and work her like a puppet on a string.

Daisy got into her car and drove away. Somewhere along the way she had lost her independence and become some lovestruck zombie following along without thinking or doing anything for herself. It should have been a relief to shake herself out of that daze but, as she drove to the cottage, the only thing she could feel was her heart splintering into a thousand sharp shards.

Even before she opened her front door, tears were blurring her vision. Time had not eased the pain of having her trust broken again. If anything, this hurt so much more. She wasn't some naïve kid who didn't know any better; she was an adult who had been burned before and had spent years making sure she didn't get herself trapped in this very scenario. It was her own fault for sharing too much, for trusting again, for falling for someone who could hurt her so easily.

Her footsteps on the bare floorboards echoed around the walls as she walked into her living room. She didn't know if it was worse seeing her belongings floating in dirty river water or finding everything gone. Her new life in Little Morton had been obliterated. Including the love and the future she'd thought she had found with Thomas. The house was empty, devoid of anything which held any meaning or sign of being loved. Exactly how she felt inside.

CHAPTER ELEVEN

EVEN WITH A houseful of patients and Daisy working in the room next door, Thomas was lonelier and unhappier than he could remember. It had been a couple of weeks since she had called it quits. He had tried to convince himself it was an inevitable outcome and he would have regretted letting her move into his home if she was capable of walking away so easily. At night, his empty house and heart said differently.

She would only speak to him on a professional basis, leaving no room for him to make apologies, though he had tried. Even then, she made sure the majority of their correspondence went through Eunice, leaving their intermediate scurrying between their offices wearing a harassed expression on her face most of the day.

He was drained emotionally and physically exhausted, kept awake at night by thoughts of how he had messed things up. If he thought Daisy would have given him another chance, he would have begged to be able to put things right again. He understood that in his enthusiasm to start a life with her he had frightened her off, but he hadn't had any sinister motive in moving her things in from the cottage. All he had wanted to do was make her comfortable in his home and prove to her that she was welcome.

Since his epic mistake, Thomas realised how inadequate he was as a partner. His distrust of strangers and his need for privacy at all costs had severely affected his ability to read what the important people in his life needed from him. He was a good doctor, but when it came to his personal life he clearly had some work to do. Not for the first time he wished his father was around to advise him. He had never had any problems expressing his feelings for Daisy and how much he liked her, and that appreciation had been mutual. Thomas could have done with a few pointers before he had lost the only woman in his life he was ever likely to love.

He didn't even know how Daisy was coping in the cottage after she had lost everything, and he was concerned she might decide to move away and start over somewhere else.

It wasn't supposed to be this way for any of them.

'Dr Ryan? Dr Swift would like to know if you could add one of her patients to your list of house calls.' Poor Eunice tentatively hovered in the doorway once his last patient had gone.

At least he had work and Daisy's presence—albeit at a distance—here to look forward to.

'Of course. Just leave me the details and I'll stop by on my rounds.' He respected Daisy's medical opinion sufficiently to not question her reasons but would have to acquaint himself with the case. Previously, she would have come in to ask him herself, perched her backside on his desk and given him the low-down on her patient while they drank their umpteenth cuppa of the day. He missed that. He would miss it more if she did resign as she had threatened to do, yet they couldn't carry on working in this atmosphere. It was painful for all involved, just having to see each other, and not see each other, every day.

He could spend all day hoping to catch the slightest glimpse of her, only to have that swell of sickness in his stomach when the sight of her reminded him that she was no longer part of his life. It felt as though she had in some way betrayed him when he had made so many changes to try and make her feel safe. Clearly he had stuffed up, but Daisy wasn't a woman who gave second chances any more. He understood that, but that didn't stop the hurt of losing her.

'Dr Ryan, there's a lady here who urgently needs help. She's not one of our patients, but I think she should really see someone.' A perturbed Eunice showed up again with a woman standing right behind her clutching her midriff and her long, lank hair seemingly matted with blood.

Thomas quickly rose to usher them inside. 'Of course. Come in.'

As he came over to welcome her in, she flinched away from him, sticking close to Eunice. Sensing her uneasiness, he stood back to let the two women into his office without crowding them.

'What's your name, love?' Eunice was the one who pulled a chair over and coaxed her into sitting down.

'Alice.'

Now he could see her better, Thomas would have said she couldn't have been any more than twenty years old. Yet, even beyond her apparent injuries, her general demeanour suggested she was someone already worn down by life.

'And your surname? Is there anyone you'd like me to call?' Alice was clearly a vulnerable person, and it would be better for her if she had someone she knew with her.

'No, I don't want anyone to know I'm here. It's just Alice.'

He and Eunice exchanged concerned looks. This was more than a simple injury. She was frightened and they would have to tread carefully in case they scared her away.

'Okay, Alice. I'm going to take a look at those nasty cuts on your face. Do you want to tell me what happened?' Thomas made sure his hands were clean before donning some surgical gloves and let Eunice comfort her while he got some cotton balls and antiseptic to clean her wounds.

'I fell.'

He didn't believe that for a moment. Especially when the injuries appeared to be on both sides of her body and he could see the shadow of an old bruise under one eye. No doubt if he questioned her about that she would tell him she had walked into a cupboard door. Excuses he had heard from victims of domestic abuse before. It sickened him to think that someone was capable of doing this to Alice.

'It must have been a bad fall to cut you like

that. If that had been any closer to your eye you might have needed surgery.' The skin above her eyebrow was split, blood trickling into the corner of her eye and down her face, but she said nothing.

Thomas went to dab at the cut but she shrank away from him, reaching out for Eunice's hand.

'Perhaps you would prefer it if Daisy, my colleague, tended to that?' He could see that she was fearful of him, and if it had been a man who had inflicted these injuries she would probably feel safer with a female doctor treating her. Despite their personal issues, he knew Daisy would want to help this young woman.

Alice nodded, suddenly tearful.

'It's fine. Don't you worry, Alice, you're safe here. I'll be back soon.' He took off his gloves and discarded them with the cotton balls to go and get Daisy's assistance. It was not unusual for female patients to request her; likewise, sometimes the men preferred to have Thomas treat them. In this instance it was important that they kept Alice calm and made her feel safe so she could get whatever help she needed after her ordeal.

He hurried next door where, thankfully, her door was open and she was sitting alone at her desk. For a split-second Thomas took in the picture of her sitting by the window, the sun creating a golden silhouette of the beautiful woman he knew he had lost his heart to. She rubbed the back of her neck, reminding him she was not some ornamental statue he had commissioned to remember her by. For now, Daisy was still here, flesh and blood, and he wondered if it was too late to fix things between them. He didn't wish to wander these halls with even more ghosts to haunt him when he was alone in the house.

'Are you going to stand there gawping all day or are you going to tell me what you want?' Daisy didn't as much as glance in his direction, yet she had known he was there.

Thomas coughed away his embarrassment at being caught staring. 'I…er…was hoping you could help me with a young woman next door. She has a head injury and possibly some damage to her ribs.'

'Shouldn't you advise her to go to the hospital?'

'I don't think she wants to be seen somewhere so public. She says she fell but there are old bruises still healing. I don't want to scare her off and I think she would be more comfortable with a female doctor.' He didn't have to say any more to get Daisy onside.

Most GPs had some experience dealing with victims of domestic violence and the most commonly used excuses.

'What's her name?' There was a grim determination in Daisy's manner now as she draped her stethoscope around her neck and walked the short distance with him.

'Alice.'

As soon as they entered his office, her demeanour changed, a smile replacing the thin-lipped expression she'd worn when Thomas had told her what he was dealing with.

'Hi, Alice. I'm Daisy, one of the GPs here. Now, Dr Ryan tells me you've had a nasty fall?' She donned a fresh pair of gloves and scooted a chair over to sit with the young woman.

Their patient nodded but she wasn't scrabbling to get away as Daisy took a look at the cut on her eye.

'Eunice? Perhaps you could go and make some hot, sweet tea and Dr Ryan and I will see to Alice.' Daisy took control of the situation, sending the receptionist away to keep anything Alice told them in confidence.

'Yes, Doctor.' The way she took off said she was only too happy to leave them to it.

Thomas sat back and let Daisy take the lead since the young woman was more likely to open up to her. He stayed in the room not only to witness anything which happened or was said, but to be here as support for Daisy. These cases were never easy, and he knew it could bring up difficult memories of the troubled relationship Daisy had told him about with her domineering ex.

'This might sting a little bit, Alice. It's quite a deep wound and I need to make sure it's clean, so infection doesn't set in.' She set to work dabbing the cut with the cotton and antiseptic, Alice wincing with the first application.

'I think you should really get that checked at the hospital. It's going to need stitches.'

'No. Can't you do it here?' The wide-eyed panic in the girl's eyes was heartbreaking when she clearly felt it wasn't safe to get the help she needed.

Daisy looked at him and he nodded before going to get the sutures to help close the wound for her.

'Alice, you seemed to be in some pain when you first came in. If you don't want to go to the hospital, maybe you would be okay with Daisy taking a look to make sure you didn't hurt yourself anywhere else when you fell?' He diverted attention away from the most obvious injury, which Daisy had now patched up, and towards the right-hand side of her body, which she clutched at every now and then.

'If you want to pop up on the bed I can pull the curtain around and give you some more privacy?' Daisy offered and Alice eventually agreed. If Thomas thought his presence here was making her unduly uncomfortable he would leave, but for now he was going to sit in to see what steps they could both take to get Alice to a place of safety.

Eunice knocked before bringing in a tray with three cups of tea and set it on the desk.

'Thanks, Eunice.'

'Is everything okay?' she mouthed back to him.

He winked and nodded, praying it would be.

In the background, Daisy was gently persuading Alice to let her examine her injuries. 'If you could take your top off, or even lift it up for me… That's great… That's a bad bruise you have there… I'm going to press gently… Let me know where it's tender…'

When Alice let out a pained yelp, Thomas winced in sympathy with her.

'The ribs are very badly bruised. I'd prefer it if you had an X-ray to make sure there's nothing broken but I will recommend you take it easy for a while. Rest up and take some painkillers.' Daisy came out from behind the curtains and pulled off the disposable gloves. A frown wrinkled her forehead and disapproval was there in the tight line of her mouth. Thomas felt the same way about whoever had caused those injuries.

Alice appeared again, pulling down her top and covering whatever injuries Daisy had been privy to.

'You know, Alice, I used to have a lot of… falls. My life was so much better once I got help and moved out of the toxic relationship I was in.'

Daisy's admission stunned Thomas and Alice into silence. He had been aware that she'd had trouble with her ex but he hadn't realised that extended to physical harm. It made his stomach knot to think of her in a similar position to Alice, broken and frightened. Not the confident, self-assured doctor who had firmly put him in his place from the moment she had arrived here.

It was difficult to marry those two versions of Daisy and he could see how hard she must have worked to get where she was today. And why she was so fiercely independent and determined to do things her way. It was her way of protecting herself from ending up in the same situation. He could relate to that when his emotional scars had caused him to shut himself off too, afraid of making the same mistakes again.

Thomas thought back to their tiff when he had accused her of overreacting to him moving her stuff in without her consent. He was such a dolt. Too caught up in what he wanted, he had been oblivious to her plight. He had taken over, disregarded her feelings and invaded her privacy. Everything she had feared by getting involved with someone again. He had shown all the signs of being another controlling partner and that was exactly why her shutters had come hurtling down, blocking him out of her life. Even if it was too late to explain his actions and accept responsibility for making her uncomfortable, Thomas would find some way of making amends so she could at least see he was not a complete monster.

Daisy was desperately attempting to hide her own emotions while she tried to cajole Alice into accepting help. She knew from experience it was not easy to make that big life change and leave that kind of relationship when it was your whole world. Being in this position, sharing her abusive past, was bringing up a lot of emotions for her too. Things she hoped she had moved past and would never have to deal with again, but recent events with Thomas had brought a lot of those unresolved issues to the fore again. It would be worth it though if she could persuade Alice to escape from her toxic relationship too, paying it forward after the help she had received from the Earl all those years ago.

'How...how did you get away?' Alice's voice was small, as though afraid to say the words aloud, and Daisy's heart went out to her and all the other women like her, still trapped with men who abused them to make themselves feel better.

'I was lucky. I heard about a lovely man who helped me. Then I went to college, studied really hard and was determined I would take care of myself from that moment on.' She could feel Thomas's eyes on her and knew this was coming as a revelation to him too.

Perhaps if she had shared more of what she had gone through they could have avoided the scene in his house altogether, but the damage was done. Even talking about her ex now made her realise Thomas was nothing like Aaron. With some space she was able to look at the two different situations and see the motives for his actions had been completely different to the man who had treated her so badly in the past. Not that it mattered now, when they had both retreated to their individual corners, clinging tightly to that emotional baggage which kept them safe from predators. At least if they could make arrangements for Alice to live independently from her abuser, something good would come out of all of this.

'Do you have any family we could call for you? Perhaps a loved one could take you in and give you somewhere to stay?' Thomas interjected. Though he meant well, family was not always the best option in these instances. They would have been the last people Daisy would have turned to for help.

'My mum would let me stay, I know she would, but I haven't seen her in so long. Arty stopped letting me call her, didn't like her coming to the house and eventually we lost contact.' Alice was shredding the tissue she had pulled from the box on Thomas's desk, her anxiety showing in every tear.

It was typical manipulative behaviour, cutting her off from anyone who might tell her to leave, convincing her that her partner was the only one who had her best interests at heart. All the while grinding her down until her confidence was at an all-time low and she didn't think she deserved any better. At least it sounded as though Alice did have a parent who loved her and might be able to get her out of her boyfriend's grasp.

'I'm sure your mother would be only too glad to hear from you. Why don't you give her a call? Or myself or Dr Swift could do it for you?' Thomas pushed his phone across the desk towards her, keen to get Alice to take that first step.

There were refuges and safe houses they could contact for her too, but if Alice had a real home to go back to it could make all the difference. Daisy almost envied her having somewhere safe she could retreat to for her recovery. She had never had anywhere except the home she had made for herself. The only time she had really felt as though someone was looking out for her was during the storm when Thomas had taken everything in hand and comforted her when she had needed it. Then she had gone and ruined everything by freaking out when he had made one kind gesture too many. Now she had nothing.

'I... I think I should be the one to call. I don't want her to worry.' Bless Alice, for thinking that her poor mother was already frightened to death for her daughter who was living with a dangerous man, capable of hurting her. Still, it would be better for her to start a dialogue now and make that connection in case she had second thoughts and thought going back would be the easier option.

'We'll give you some privacy, but we'll just be outside the door if you need us.' Thomas rose from his chair and Daisy followed him out into the hallway.

They stood awkwardly together, not really knowing what to say to each other. It was Thomas who finally made the first move.

'That must have been hard for you in there.'

She swallowed down the sudden ball of emotion trying to block her airway. 'It was important Alice knew she had someone she could confide in. Who wouldn't judge her or tell her she'd been stupid to put up with it for so long. It's not as easy to get out of a situation like that as people think.'

'You really helped get through to her. Hopefully this will get her the help she needs.'

'I hope so too.'

Thomas had been right to come to her for help in the first place. Some might have turned Alice away. Daisy remembered plucking up the courage to go and see a doctor once, not knowing where else to go. He'd accused her of wasting his time and being a silly little girl. It was an age before she'd even contemplated asking for help again.

Thomas was compassionate to anyone in need, and she could only conclude that the dark light she had cast him in recently was mostly down to her own issues. Yes, he had overstepped the mark, but it was a mistake he had tried to apologise for repeatedly. She was the one who'd continued to hold a grudge because it was safer than admitting she had fallen for him. A good excuse for her to keep her distance instead of letting the relationship blossom and put her heart on the line for him. Even though Thomas already unwittingly held it in his hands.

That realisation had freaked her out more than his interference in her living arrangements and deep down she knew that was why she had run out on him. What she had to decide now was whether or not she wanted to stay in Little Morton, pull up her big girl pants and tell him how she felt, or keep running away from those feelings. Should she open her heart or protect it at all costs?

'Daisy, I had no idea you'd gone through so much yourself. I'm truly sorry if my actions brought you more pain. That was not my intention.'

'I know,' she conceded. 'I should never even

have joked about moving in. I guess we could call it a mutual misunderstanding.' Letting him continue to think the whole debacle was his fault wouldn't be fair to Thomas when they had both made mistakes.

Before they could discuss the matter any further or consider what this meant for them now, Alice opened the office door.

'Mum says I can go and stay with her,' she said with a heartbreaking smile. It must have come as such a relief and a revelation to know she was still wanted and loved, despite any disagreements in the past.

Daisy longed for the same. Would Thomas accept her half-apology and be willing to try again when she had hurt him so cruelly by walking away when he had made room in his life for her? Was that what she even wanted? On her part at least the answer was yes, but she couldn't be one hundred per cent sure she was brave enough to take that step again.

'That's fantastic, Alice.'

'That's the first step. I'm so pleased for you.' Daisy agreed with Thomas's sentiment. This was the best news they could have hoped for.

'I hate to ask but I might need to borrow my bus fare. Mum doesn't drive and I don't have any money. I don't want her to see me like this. Maybe I should go back and get some of my things…' Alice glanced at her bloodstained shirt and Daisy could see why she was worried, but going back for any reason was a bad idea. Making the break was the biggest step and there was no way of knowing what she could be returning to in that house.

'Listen, Alice, if there is nothing really important back there, I would walk away. I can drive you wherever you need to be and we can stop and get you a change of clothes on the way.' Someone had stepped up to help Daisy start over and she would be only too happy to do the same for Alice.

'I could come with you too…or just give you my credit card to get whatever Alice needs…' Halfway through his offer Thomas seemed to have a change of heart, no doubt afraid he was overstepping the mark again. Daisy appreciated that he wanted to support them both, especially if there was a violent partner involved, but there was no need. As she had to keep reminding herself, she wasn't the helpless young girl she had once been. Hopefully the same would soon be said about Alice too.

'Thanks, Thomas, but I think we can manage. Besides, you will need to hold the fort here.' She gave him a smile to convey her thanks, that there was no ill feeling on her part, and hoped the same was true for him.

'No problem. You know where I am if you need me.' Thomas walked away, leaving her and Alice to fend for themselves, just as Daisy had asked him to.

If she had made it clear from the beginning what she did or did not need from him they would likely still be together. All Thomas had done was try to make her feel a part of something, even if he had gone about it the wrong way. The notion of sharing her life again had terrified her. Thinking the worst about Thomas's well-intended gesture had given her a good reason to back away. She hadn't known what she would do if the same happened again somewhere down the line, if forgiving one transgression left the door open for more to occur. So Daisy had taken the easy option and retreated back into her safe, lonely shell.

The problem was she had enjoyed being with Thomas and could picture them as a couple. If she hadn't screwed things up with him altogether, she had to decide once and for all if she was willing to trust, to love again, or let the bad guys win by continuing to live alone and miserable.

* * *

Daisy had to struggle to focus on the road. Dealing with Alice had brought back so many bad memories for her to deal with she was exhausted. Plus there were no streetlights on the lane back to her cottage. Not that she was in a rush to get home. There was nothing waiting for her there except empty rooms and memories of Thomas and everything she had turned away from.

She yawned as she drew up towards the cottage and was forced to slam the brakes on when she nearly ran into the car parked outside.

'What the hell?' An unexpected visitor was the last thing she wanted to deal with tonight.

A cold chill ran in her veins when she considered the possibility that it could be Alice's partner come looking for her. He might have heard she had been at the clinic and hunted Daisy down to find out what had happened and where she had gone. With Alice gone, he might take out his frustrations on her.

She grabbed her bag but her phone was dead and the only thing inside she could use as a weapon was a compact umbrella. Armed with her makeshift cudgel, she got out of her car and walked tentatively towards the dark figure sitting in the car in her driveway.

Just as she was getting ready to make vague threats against the intruder, on closer inspection she realised it was Thomas slumped in the front seat. He was fast asleep, his breath steaming against the window. If he was waiting for her he could have let himself into the cottage until she came home, but he probably hadn't wanted to risk her wrath again by intruding onto the property. Knowing she couldn't leave him out here in the cold all night, Daisy rapped on the glass.

'Thomas? Come in out of the cold.'

He startled then saw her, smiled and got out of the car clutching a manila folder.

'How long have you been sitting out here?'

'A couple of hours. You weren't answering your phone and I wanted to make sure everything went well with Alice.' He followed her into the cottage as she turned on the lights and the central heating.

'A couple of hours? You must be freezing and out of your mind.' Although she was touched he had waited that long to make sure she was okay.

Thomas shrugged. 'I realised what dealing with Alice meant to you and couldn't stop thinking about everything you must have suffered in the past.'

Daisy shuddered, trying not to think about

it too much and focus on Alice's progress. 'I've tried to put it behind me but sometimes it does sneak up on me. I'm sorry if I transferred some of those residual issues onto you. As for Alice, it all looks promising so far. We got her some clean clothes and drove to her mum's. Naturally she was over the moon to have her daughter back and managed to talk Alice into going to the hospital for a check-up, telling her to get it on record. The ribs were just bruised, as we suspected, so she should make a quick recovery.'

'I'm glad. I was thinking that perhaps we could look into setting up a charity to help other women in similar situations.'

'I would love that; it's a great idea. We could fund a safe house and help get them into employment, so they would be working towards their independence.' She'd got a buzz helping Alice break away today and it would give her a real sense of purpose to help desperate women make a new start. Thomas's father would have approved too, she was sure.

'Does that mean you're staying?'

'I think so.' She was content here. It was only the ghosts of her past which continued to make her miserable. Daisy guessed that would go on for as long as she let it. It was about time she took back control and dictated her own happiness. That included having Thomas in her life.

'In that case, you might need these.' He handed over the folder he had tucked under his arm. When Daisy opened it she found legal documents relating to the cottage.

'What's this?'

'The deeds to the cottage. I want you to be comfortable here, and if that means giving you this place, so be it. I know my father would have wanted you to have this anyway.'

'I would never have accepted it off him either. I told you I never came here with any ulterior motive. I simply loved your father for the special man he was. The male role model I never had in my life.'

'It was stupid of me to say those things about you at the festival. I don't think you came here for his money, but I do want you to have the cottage. It's your home. You don't owe me anything in return and it will give you peace of mind that I will never set foot in here again without your permission.'

Daisy was speechless. Not only was this an unbelievable gift but it was a spectacular display of trust on his part. If she was so inclined, she could sell the cottage and do a runner. He was willing to risk that sort of betrayal again in the hope she would stick around. Even if he didn't know it himself, only a man who truly loved her would take that sort of chance. Thomas deserved the same recognition in return when Daisy knew she had fallen in love with him from that first day, when he had carried her shoes and handbag without saying a word.

'There's really no need to do this, Thomas.'

'There's every need when I want you to stay. You mean the world to me, Daisy. I know I messed things up between us and I'll understand if you can never forgive me for that. I just want you to know I wasn't trying to take over, or make you feel insignificant. It was my stupid way of showing you I cared. Maybe I should have just told you I loved you and saved all the trouble.' He mumbled the last bit as he turned back towards the door.

If Daisy let him leave now she knew she would lose him for ever. This was the time for her to have a say in what was going to happen next in her life. She had to make that move forward or remain stagnant for the rest of her days.

'Thomas, wait.' She reached for his hand and pulled him back towards her. He looked at her hand then at her face with such hope in his eyes Daisy's heart gave an extra flutter.

'Say that again. The bit where you muttered something about loving me.'

'I love you, Daisy, and if you'll let me I'll spend the rest of my days proving it to you.'

'I think you've already done that. There is such a thing as overkill, you know.' She smiled at him and saw the relief on his face that she was finally hearing him out.

Thomas smiled back. 'As long as you don't hate me any more.'

'I could never hate you. What on earth would make you think that?' Daisy took the bold move of slipping her arms around his waist, hoping an embrace wasn't too much to expect after everything.

'I don't know. Maybe it was the not speaking to me for what seemed like for ever, or perhaps it was when you said you wanted a transfer.' Thankfully Thomas appeared to have forgiven her for her past transgressions as he took her in his arms.

'I'm sorry. I got it all wrong. I know you would never hurt me. I was confused about how I was feeling and afraid everything was going to go wrong again. It was easier for me to run away from it all than face it.'

'And now? How do you feel about me? About us?' Thomas bent his head so his mouth was hovering a mere whisper away from hers, waiting for her permission to close that tiny gap.

'I love you, Thomas Ryan. I love us and I want to try again.'

'That's all I needed to hear.' He set his mouth on hers and kissed her so gently Daisy knew she had made the right decision. Thomas was someone who would take care of her the way no one else in her life ever had.

She had finally decided to take a chance on her Prince Charming and she prayed they would both get their happy-ever-after.

EPILOGUE

One year later

'ARE YOU FINISHED in there?' Thomas called through the bathroom door, waiting for Daisy to come out.

'Patience is not your strong point, is it, my darling?' She put him out of his misery by coming out to join him in the bedroom.

'No? I'm still waiting for you to accept my marriage proposal, aren't I?' He sat down on the bed and patted the space beside him. Daisy went to him, clutching the pregnancy test in her hand that he was so desperate to see, even though they wouldn't know the result for another few minutes.

'That's marriage proposals, plural.' It had become something of a standing joke between them now that he would get down on one knee at any given opportunity and ask her to marry him, even though she had said no every time.

'I live in hope that one day you will say yes and make me the happiest man in the world.'

Despite the fact that she had moved in with him several months ago to show how serious she was about the relationship, Daisy had not been ready to go all in and get wed. She was still clinging onto her independence and she had no idea why, other than that residual fear that she would be handing over control of her life to someone who might abuse that trust. It was ridiculous when Thomas had proved repeatedly that he was nothing like the men who had hurt her in the past.

After getting it so very wrong by moving her things in without telling her, he had made a conscious effort since to ensure she was comfortable with every step they took as a couple, consulting her about each room in the house as he'd begun to make the place into a home for them both. He had redecorated and sold a lot of the family heirlooms to fund the safe house they had created for vulnerable women at the cottage.

She couldn't have asked for a more considerate partner. He told her he loved her every day, showed her that in his every action, and she knew he would never have asked her to move in if it wasn't the truth. Of course she loved him with every fibre of her being too and couldn't imagine life without him now. There was just that one hurdle to get over...

'What if the test is positive?' she asked. They hadn't planned to have a baby so early on in their relationship, but they had not been as careful as they should have been where contraception was concerned. Daisy liked to think it was an unacknowledged part of their commitment and trust that if she did fall pregnant they would both step up and be there for one another, as they always had been.

'Then I will be absolutely over the moon. I never thought I would be a father and the chance to raise a family with you feels like I'm in a dream. I had a great relationship with my father, and I hope for the same with my own children. This baby would have a happy, loving home with two parents who will want only the very best for him or her.' He was already beaming at the prospect and Daisy knew he would be a great dad when he had so much love to give. They had both grown up in a broken home, so they knew how important it was for a child to feel safe and happy.

When they had done so much soul-searching before committing to their relationship, Daisy was positive Thomas was 'the one' she was going to share the rest of her life with. Which begged the question why she hadn't agreed to be his wife yet. A piece of paper wasn't going to change anything except to give them that sense of belonging. Her heart and soul were already Thomas's and accepting his surname wasn't going to suddenly turn him into the controlling monster she feared. Being his wife didn't necessarily mean she would be giving anything up, but she would be gaining a family in him and any children they might be lucky enough to have.

'What if I'm not pregnant?' It was one thing contemplating marriage knowing there was a baby on the way and wanting to 'do the right thing', but if this was a false alarm she was afraid the disappointment would overshadow the engagement she was now contemplating.

'Then we can try again when we're ready. It won't change the way I feel about you, Daisy. I love you and I'm yours for ever.'

Every time he said the words he claimed another piece of her heart and made her fall in love with him even more. She was only hurting them both by refusing his offer of marriage when it would cement their relationship for ever.

'Ask me the question.' Right now she was surer than she had ever been that this was what she wanted. Thomas. A family. Even if she wasn't pregnant now, she hoped that some day they would be looking forward to the arrival of their child. In the meantime she was happy to put the past behind her and focus on the future she could have with Thomas.

'*The* question? Why, when I already know the answer?'

She gave him *the look* which he knew meant there was no point in arguing. Thomas was no doormat, but he would do absolutely anything for her. That worked both ways, which was why they had such a great relationship. They were a team, at work and at home. Hopefully as parents too.

He sighed but still got down on one knee and took her hand. 'Daisy Swift, would you do me the absolute honour of being my wife?'

'Yes.' She beamed, enjoying the complete shock registering on his face.

'Really? This isn't a wind-up?'

'No,' she said, laughing. 'I love you, Thomas Ryan, and I can't wait to be your wife.'

'You won't have to wait. Name the day and I'll be there waiting at the end of the aisle for you.' He hugged her and kissed her hard on the lips. Daisy was the happiest she had ever been in her life and there was just one more thing that would make everything perfect.

'Time's up. Should we take a look at the results?' She opened up her hand to check the plastic window which would reveal if they were going to be parents soon or if they would have to wait a little longer.

They were both holding their breath as they checked the results.

'Positive.' Thomas confirmed what she had seen for herself but didn't quite believe it.

'We're going to be parents,' she said aloud as it began to sink in.

'We're going to be a family.' Thomas was clutching her hands, his eyes filled with happy tears, and Daisy finally knew what it was to be loved.

It was everything.

* * * * *

*If you enjoyed this story, check out
these other great reads from
Karin Baine*

Wed for Their One Night Baby
The Nurse's Christmas Hero
The Surgeon and the Princess
One Night with Her Italian Doc

All available now!